Chair Exercises for Seniors

Your 28-Day Plan to Enhanced Strength and Independence - An Illustrated, Step-by-Step Guide with 80+ Seated Exercises

Free Bonuses from Scott Hamrick available for limited time

Hi seniors!

My name is Scott Hamrick, and first off, I want to THANK YOU for reading my book.

Now you have a chance to join my exclusive "workout for seniors" email list so you can get the ebook below for free as well as the potential to get more ebooks for seniors for free! Simply click the link below to join.

P.S. Remember that it's 100% free to join the list.

Access your free bonuses here

https://livetolearn.lpages.co/chair-exercises-for-seniors-28-day-paperback/

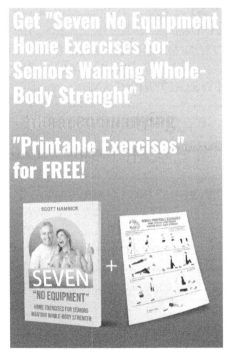

Or, Scan the QR code!

Table of Contents

Introduction

Are you looking to improve your physical health and well-being with chair exercises? Do you want to watch your muscles work while chilling on a chair? Are you new to chair exercises? Are you looking for simple yet effective exercises that you can engage in? If your answer is a resounding yes or even an unsure maybe, you picked the right book.

Did you know? Chair exercises are fantastic for improving your health and fitness without straining your body. These exercises are performed while sitting or holding onto a chair for support. They offer a gentle way to increase strength, flexibility, and balance. For older adults who may have mobility issues or find traditional exercise routines challenging, chair exercises provide a safe and accessible option to stay active and maintain your overall well-being.

Chair exercises offer a ton of benefits. They help improve joint mobility, which is especially beneficial for individuals with arthritis or other age-related joint issues. Chair exercises also help enhance balance and coordination, reducing the risk of falls — a common concern among older adults. These exercises can help alleviate stiffness, increase circulation, and promote better posture, contributing to overall physical comfort and confidence in daily activities.

This book is specifically tailored for seniors of all fitness levels, offering a comprehensive guide to chair exercises that is easy to follow and understand. But what sets this book apart from others on the market? The step-by-step instructions provided in this manual are designed with seniors in mind, focusing on simplicity and clarity to ensure maximum effectiveness and safety. It is designed to show seniors like you how to do these seated exercises safely and effectively with a complete plan laid out for 28 days. Whether you're new to exercise or looking to maintain your strength and independence as you age, this book offers something for everyone. They're not just any exercises — they're meant to make you stronger and help you move better.

One unique feature of this book is its emphasis on promoting independence and strength in seniors. The exercises included are carefully selected to target key muscle groups and functional movements, helping older adults maintain their ability to perform activities of daily living with ease and confidence. By incorporating these exercises into your routine, you can enhance your quality of life and enjoy greater freedom and mobility as you age.

With this guide in your hands, you'll have everything you need to embark on a journey toward better health and vitality through chair exercises. Are you ready to achieve all your fitness goals and live life to the fullest?

Chapter 1: Foundations First: Embracing Chair Exercises

Exercise is vital for people of all ages. When one gets older, it goes beyond getting in shape and losing weight. Physical activity becomes a necessity as it slows down many age-related health problems. Many seniors lose their independence and start relying on others to help them with their basic needs. Exercising strengthens the muscles so you can perform your daily tasks without assistance.

However, physical activities don't come easy for all seniors. Some lack flexibility, while others suffer from balance and coordination issues, which make working out challenging. Luckily, chair exercises consider older adults' physical limitations. They can provide you with the same benefits as regular exercises and suit different fitness levels and mobility capabilities.

This chapter introduces chair exercises, their significance, and how they can address age-related physical issues.

What Are Chair Exercises?

Chair or sitting exercises are alternative forms of physical activity that you can perform on a regular chair or a wheelchair. They target different parts of the body and promote physical fitness. These exercises are suitable for older adults and people with mobility issues.

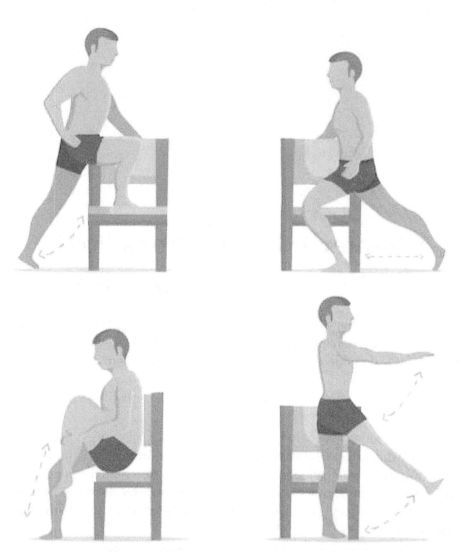

Chair exercises are alternative forms of physical activity that you can perform on a regular chair. *Designed by Freepik. https://www.freepik.com/free-vector/rehabilitation-exercises-with-chair_1196186.htm#fromView=search&page=2&position=47&uuid=b4d55a79-25d5-4288-b6ff-677b48403137*

Exercising is vital for health. However, aging and many health issues make the lives of older adults difficult, and many struggle to lead normal and independent lives.

Chair exercises can benefit people suffering from a wide range of health conditions:

- Neurological disorders

- Cognitive disorders
- Physical disabilities
- Spinal cord injuries
- Dementia
- Alzheimer's
- Parkinson's disease
- Strokes
- Type 2 diabetes
- High blood pressure
- Osteoarthritis

The Significance of Chair Exercises for Older Adults

Although chair exercises can benefit people of all ages and health conditions, they are particularly beneficial to older adults. They are effective workouts that target the core muscles, legs, and arms without the need to get out of your chair. This reduces the risk of falling and injury in people with mobility and balance issues.

According to a 2016 study conducted by the University of Manchester, older adults who regularly practice chair exercises show great improvements in their cognitive skills and are noticeably in a better mood. According to a 2020 study conducted by the University of Coimbra, Portugal, chair exercises have a huge impact on older women's physical health, and they reduce their risk of falling.

In another 2020 study conducted by Kumamoto Rehabilitation Hospital in Japan, chair exercises can improve swallowing ability in people recovering from stroke. These people are also able to return to their regular lives and perform their daily activities quickly.

Physical Challenges for Older Adults

Older adults face many physical challenges with age. Half of these issues are associated with a lack of physical activity.

Low Muscle Mass

People start to lose muscle mass in their 30s. By the time they turn 60, they will have lost over 10%, and this will accelerate between the ages of 65 and 75. Physically inactive individuals lose more muscle mass than people who regularly exercise. This loss reduces mobility and muscle strength.

Loss of muscle mass affects your ability to perform your daily activities and tasks with ease and reduces your quality of life. As a result, you may lose your independence and require full-time care. It also affects your body's skeletal system, which is responsible for mobility and protecting your organs. This increases the risk of frailty, falls, and fractures.

Symptoms of muscle-mass loss include loss of stamina, weakness, walking slowly, decrease in muscle size, imbalance, higher risk of falling, decrease in physical endurance, and difficulty climbing stairs.

How Can Chair Exercises Help?

Chair exercises work on improving handgrip strength and arm curl performance, which can build muscles and increase strength and independence.

Coordination and Balance Issues

Aging also affects coordination. Your nervous system is responsible for keeping you coordinated so you can easily perform daily activities without falling or losing your balance. For example, you will be able to carry your cup of coffee across the room without dropping it.

Due to a lack of diet and poor exercise, older adults suffer from ministrokes that usually go unnoticed but can affect the parts of the brain responsible for coordination.

Aging also impacts your balance due to changes in your blood pressure, poor circulation, neurological diseases, side effects of medication, and low blood sugar and iron levels.

Symptoms of lack of coordination and balance include trouble swallowing, uncontrollable eye movement, change in speech, unsteadiness, confusion, blurred vision, disorientation, and dizziness.

How Can Chair Exercises Help?

Chair exercises target your lower body and enhance your balance. They also strengthen your legs, hips, and core, reduce the risk of falls and injuries, and improve your coordination.

Regular exercises usually involve standing and performing certain movements that can be hard and risky for people suffering from coordination or mobility issues. For instance, if you can't maintain your balance, you may fall and injure yourself while working out on a treadmill.

With chair exercises, you practice in a chair, so there is less chance of getting dizzy or losing balance.

Lack of Flexibility

People become less flexible with age due to loss of muscle elasticity, stiffness in the joints, and loss of water in the spine and tissues. Lack of flexibility impacts your functional abilities, causing severe limitations to your movements. For instance, you may struggle with getting off the floor, so you avoid certain physical activities. This can affect your quality of life and cause further loss of flexibility.

How Can Chair Exercises Help?

Chair exercises usually involve stretching that strengthens the thighs and hips, improving your mobility and flexibility.

Chair exercises are effective in dealing with many age-related physical issues. They stand out from other types of physical activities because they are safe and accessible.

Unlike many other types of exercises that require equipment or a gym membership, you will only need a chair. So, you have the freedom to perform these exercises in your home, outdoors, or at a friend's or a family member's house.

Seated exercises are also adaptable, so people of all ages and activity levels can practice them.

Core Principles of Chair Exercises

Chair exercises involve slow and controlled movements, posture alignment, and muscle engagement. They are the core principles of this workout, and each one has its benefits and impact on the body.

Slow and Controlled Movements

One of the most common misconceptions is that only intense exercises that involve fast movements can be effective. This is one of the reasons why many older adults don't exercise. However, the slow and controlled movements in chair exercises have many benefits, such as burning calories, building strength, protecting you from injury, and building muscle mass.

Have you ever watched someone doing push-ups? Their movements are usually fast-paced and based on momentum. However, if they slow down, their muscles will be doing all the work, pushing them up and lowering them.

In other words, physics does all the work instead of the muscles. Slowing down and controlling your movements force you to apply all your strength in each movement, allowing you to exercise your muscles and strengthen them.

Similarly, in chair exercises, slowing down your tempo tenses the muscles for longer periods, which improves productivity and endurance.

Slow movements allow you to fully use your joints, increasing your strength and mobility.

Quick movements don't allow you to focus and improve your techniques since you are moving fast and aren't paying attention to the small details. When you practice slow and controlled movements, you will be able to spot any weaknesses or issues in your performance so you can fix them.

Chair exercises also prevent injuries because slow and controlled movements keep you focused on your technique, so you are less likely to make mistakes and hurt yourself.

Posture Alignment

Proper posture is sitting or standing upright so that your ankles, knees, hips, spine, shoulders, and head are lined up with each other, creating an alignment. This protects you against muscle strain and injuries and keeps you active. Having an ideal posture prevents kyphosis (curving of the spine), which can increase the risk of spine injuries and broken bones.

Your posture changes with age. You may struggle with standing up straight, and your spine will start to curve, resembling the top of a question mark, which people call a "hunchback." This can cause mild discomfort for some people, while in others, it can cause balance issues, shoulder, neck, and back strain, increased risk of falls, breathing problems, and loss of strength and flexibility, impacting their quality of life.

The benefits of posture alignment are:

- Good posture keeps your organs aligned and prevents them from squeezing the intestines, liver, and stomach. As a result, your body won't feel compressed, allowing for food and other fluids to flow through it. Poor posture can prevent the gastrointestinal system from performing properly, causing Gastroesophageal reflux disease and other stomach diseases.

- Poor posture stresses the muscles, causing severe discomfort. Proper posture doesn't apply any tension to the muscles or cause pain.
- Proper posture improves your balance and reduces the risk of falls, which are the main causes of injury among older adults. When you are aware of your posture, you will be more balanced and less likely to fall and injure yourself.
- Alignment prevents dropping heads and slumping shoulders, which add tension to the muscles and cause severe headaches.
- Poor posture can cause osteoarthritis (a degenerative joint disease) and osteoporosis (a condition that weakens the bones) due to the tension applied to the muscles, leading to spine degeneration.
- Proper posture allows the blood to flow properly throughout the body, preventing hypertension and protecting against strokes, obesity, heart attacks, and diabetes.
- When your spine is aligned, it supports communication between the brain and neurotransmitters, improving your memory and other cognitive functions.
- Proper posture improves blood circulation, allowing oxygen to flow through the body and improving perceptions and mood.
- Sitting and standing up straight can boost your confidence and energy levels.

One of the first steps in every chair exercise is to sit up in a proper posture. If you have a curved spine, you will start to notice a difference with regular training. However, any type of improvement takes time and effort, so be patient with yourself.

Muscle Engagement

Muscle engagement involves contracting the muscles until they become stiff enough to support the pelvis and spine. This principle aims to protect the spine and pelvis from excessive motion that occurs when you walk, bend, or pick up a child.

Muscle engagement creates stability, strengthens your body, and improves your endurance, allowing seniors to gain their independence.

They will be able to carry groceries, climb the stairs, walk, and perform daily tasks without assistance.

Engaging the muscles strengthens the joints, which improves stability and reduces osteoarthritis symptoms. It also improves balance and protects you against falls and injuries.

Bone density decreases with age, increasing the risk of fractures and osteoporosis. Chair exercises that engage the muscles strengthen the bones and improve their health.

Other Benefits of Muscle Engagement:

- Rebuilding muscle tissues in older adults.
- Boosting energy and increasing metabolism.
- Reducing fats and promoting weight loss.
- Lowering blood pressure.
- Raising the levels of HDL cholesterol (the good type) and reducing LDL cholesterol (the bad type).
- Accelerating the recovery of people suffering from cardiovascular diseases.
- Improving insulin sensitivity and aid in weight loss, reducing the risk of Type-2 diabetes.
- Helping people in wheelchairs regain physical abilities, fitness, and strength so they can walk and perform daily tasks without assistance.
- Improving mental health by reducing tension and fatigue.

Chair exercises engage the muscles, allowing you to reap all these benefits.

Basic Exercises

You are probably wondering, "How can I perform chair exercises?" This part provides basic and simple exercises to familiarize you with the format. You will be introduced to more complex routines in the coming chapters.

You should be seated in an upright position in all these exercises.

Toe Lifts

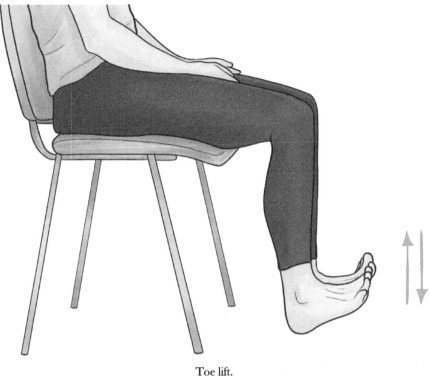

Toe lift.

Instructions:

1. Sit in an upright position with your knees together and your feet on the floor.

2. With your heels on the floor, slowly lift the toes on both feet.

3. Then, lower your toes onto the floor and lift your heels while gently squeezing your calf muscles.

4. Repeat a few times.

Overhead Press

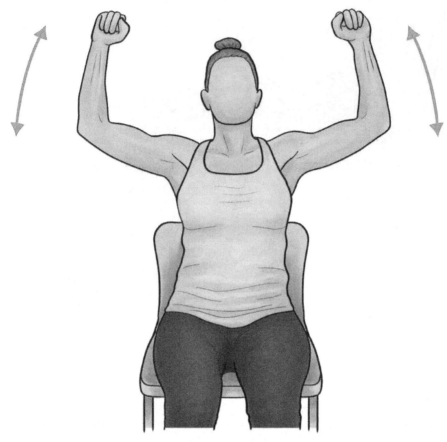

Overhead Press.

Instructions:

1. Bend your arms up so your wrists are at shoulder level.
2. In a slow and controlled movement, punch your right arm up.
3. Repeat the exercise a few times.

Chest Stretch

Chest stretch.

Instructions:

1. Sit in an upright position, but keep your back slightly away from the chair.
2. Pull your shoulder back and down.
3. Extend both arms to your sides.
4. Slowly push your chest forward until you feel a stretch in your chest.
5. Hold this position for ten seconds.
6. Repeat five times.

Seated Side Stretch

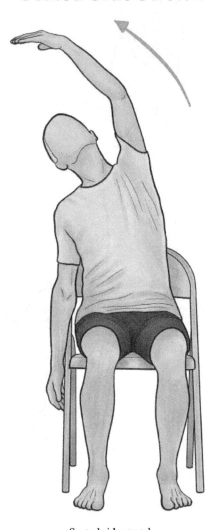

Seated side stretch

Instructions:

1. Hold tight to the right side of your chair with your right hand.
2. Extend your left arm over your head, making a shape that resembles the letter "C."
3. Shift your upper torso to the right.
4. Hold this position for 20 seconds.
5. Switch sides and repeat a few times.

Biceps Curls

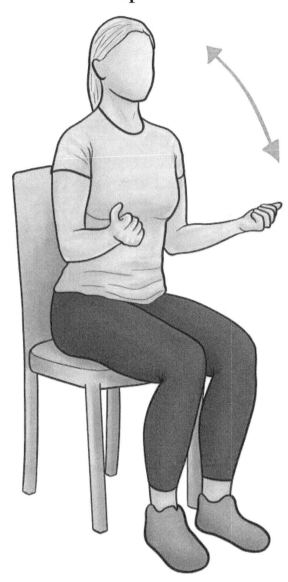

Biceps Curls.

Instructions:

1. Lift both arms at a 90-degree angle.
2. Raise and lower your forearms.
3. Repeat a few times.

Sitting to Standing

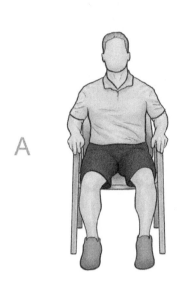
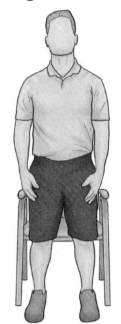

Sitting to standing.

Instructions:

1. Sit and stand using your body weight.
2. Repeat a few times.

Chin Tucks

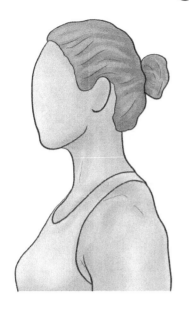 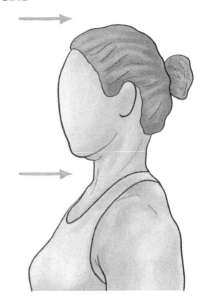

A   B

Chin tucks.

Instructions:

1. Look straight ahead.
2. Pull your chin down toward your chest.
3. Hold this position for five seconds.
4. Release, then repeat.

Ankle Rotations

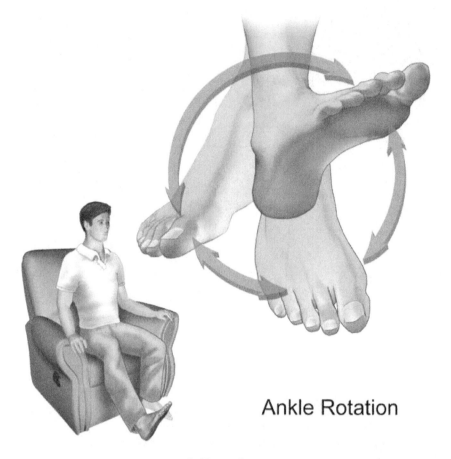

Ankle Rotation

Ankle rotation.

Instructions:

1. Place the ankle of your right foot onto your left knee.
2. Rotate your ankle in circles ten times clockwise and ten times counterclockwise.
3. Point your toes out to stretch.
4. Repeat with your left ankle.

Seated Pedaling

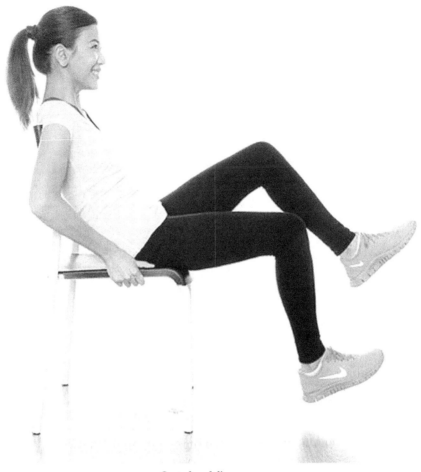

Seated pedaling.

Instructions:

1. Lift your feet as if you are pedaling.
2. Pedal for 10 to 20 minutes.

Shoulder Rolls

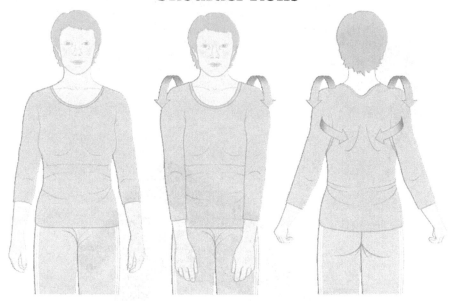

Shoulder rolls.

Instructions:

1. Sit with both feet flat on the ground.
2. Shrug your shoulders up toward your ears.
3. Slowly and gently rotate your shoulders in a circular position a few times.
4. Repeat ten times.

Tips Before Starting Exercising

- Check with a healthcare professional before starting exercising.
- Choose a stable and solid chair.
- Avoid chairs with wheels.
- Avoid chairs with arms unless the exercise requires you to use one.
- Place your chair against the wall to increase its stability.

- Sit in an upright position with your knees bent at a right angle and your feet placed flat on the floor in every exercise unless you are instructed otherwise.
- Keep a bottle of water next to you.
- Wear comfortable and loose clothes.
- Start with simple exercises and gradually increase the intensity.
- Increase repetition when your body adapts to the exercise routine.
- If an exercise makes you feel uncomfortable, stop right away and find a new one.
- Take breaks and listen to your body.
- Don't work yourself too hard.

Benefits of Chair Exercises

Chair exercises can have a huge impact on your physical and mental health. After starting an exercise routine, you will feel its impact on every area of your life.

Reduces Pain

Chair exercises improve mobility, which reduces pain. Physical activities release endorphins, which are natural painkillers. They reduce inflammation and increase joint lubrication, improving motion and reducing pain. These exercises also strengthen your core, relieving muscle tension and strain and protecting your back and shoulder from pressure and pain.

Easy on Hips and Knees

Older adults suffering from hip and knee pain can easily practice chair routines because they don't apply pressure on the joints or involve lifting weights. These exercises don't cause pain or injuries, making them ideal for older citizens.

Ideal for People with Balance Issues and Vertigo

If you suffer from low blood pressure, vertigo, or any balance-related issue, you can easily perform chair exercises without worrying about losing your balance and falling.

No Choreographed Routine

Older adults with coordination issues don't prefer choreographed routines because they struggle with memorizing the steps. They also find moving around the room to be challenging. With chair exercises, participants can be comfortable practicing in the same spot without worrying about coordination and moving their arms and legs around.

Suitable for People with Sight and Hearing Issues

Chair routines are safe for people with hearing and sight issues. Unlike running, hiking, or exercises that involve equipment, seated training protects them from accidents and injuries. The movements are also simple, so people suffering from hearing issues will be able to understand the instructor just by watching them.

They Are Easy

Some people don't like physical activity and prefer to sit on their couch and watch TV. With chair routines, even the least active people can still exercise. You don't need to leave your chair or turn off the TV. You can achieve the dream of working out while sitting down.

Versatility

Chair exercises are versatile, and you can customize them to your needs. Change the frequency, intensity, and duration to fit your preferences, needs, and activity levels. There are various exercises to choose from that target every area of the body, such as the neck, core, back, legs, arms, and chest. You can also perform these exercises with Pilates, yoga, or any other physical activity.

Sociable and Fun

Chair exercises can be fun, and you can combine them with any of your favorite hobbies. You can practice while listening to music, talking on the phone, or watching TV. You can make these exercises a sociable experience by inviting friends over to practice together or joining an exercise group in your neighborhood.

Arrange the chairs in a circle so all participants will be facing each other and so you can catch up, chat, and have fun. Unlike other exercises, there is no harm in engaging in conversation or performing other activities because there is no risk of tripping and falling.

They Boost your Self-Esteem

Many of the aging side-effects, like the risk of falling and loss of independence, can impact your self-esteem. Chair exercises help you lead a normal life, which can boost your confidence.

Chair routines are for everyone. No matter what your age, gender, or physical activity level is, you can still practice these exercises. They are easy and fun, have many health benefits, and include a variety of techniques, so you can change your routine whenever you get bored.

Don't give up if you don't notice improvement right away. You are adopting a new lifestyle for your health and well-being. Even if you don't start getting flexible or more independent in the first few months, that's okay. You are still improving other areas of your life and becoming more active.

If you feel pain while exercising, stop right away. Your body is telling you to slow down and take a break.

You will discover more exercises in this book that target every part of your body and cater to your different physical needs. You will also find mindful techniques to connect your body and mind.

Exercising isn't enough without proper hydration and nutrition. You will also find tips on preparing well-balanced meals for a healthy lifestyle.

Now that you have learned about chair exercises and familiarized yourself with their format and routine, you are ready to begin your exercise plan. Head to the next chapter for a 28-day exercise program that will increase your strength and independence.

Chapter 2: 28 Days to Greater Strength: Daily Routines

Exercising isn't a hobby that you practice in your free time. It is a necessity, and you should treat it as a priority. Nowadays, life is hectic and fast-paced. Whether young or old adults, they don't feel like they have time for self-care. However, nothing is more significant than your well-being. Make time to practice chair exercises daily, even for just a few minutes.

This chapter provides you with a 28-day plan that introduces a new chair exercise every day to improve your independence and strength.

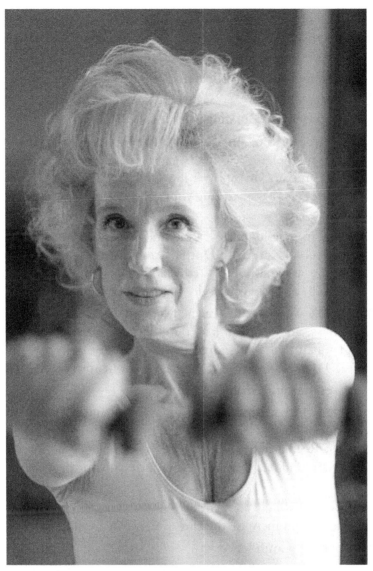
Nothing is more significant than your well-being.
https://www.pexels.com/photo/an-elderly-woman-holding-dumbbells-7927939/

The Importance of Regular Exercise

You can only reap the benefits of chair exercises when you practice a few days a week. Regular exercise helps you manage your weight, improve your mood, boost your energy, enhance your memory, reduce pain, and promote relaxation and better sleep. It also reduces the risk of many serious physical and mental health conditions like cancer, type-2 diabetes, cardiovascular disease, hypertension, LDL cholesterol, strokes, falls, arthritis, high blood pressure, anxiety, and depression.

Regular exercise also has a huge impact on your muscles, mobility, and confidence.

Regular Exercises and Building Muscles

Exercising three or four times a week can help increase your strength. After working out, your muscle fibers get damaged, which is why you feel sore. Your body repairs or replaces these fibers, increasing muscle mass. Although this process occurs during your rest time, it can't happen without physical activity.

The words "muscle damage" shouldn't worry or scare you. It is a necessary step to build strength. During exercise, you apply stress on your body by adding weights or by constantly changing your routine to challenge yourself, push your muscles harder, and damage more fibers.

Going a week without physical activity can decrease muscle strength and muscle mass, and you will lose the effects of exercise on your body. This doesn't mean that you should work out every day. Your body still needs to rest. Try not to go over three days without any physical activity.

Regular Exercises and Mobility

Nothing has a bigger impact on your mobility and independence than physical activities. They strengthen your bones and muscles and improve joint functions. Regular exercise improves your balance and strength and reduces the risk of falling. This helps you perform your daily activities with ease.

Lack of exercise affects your strength and reduces your mobility. Being physically inactive can increase the risk of disability in older adults.

Boosts Your Self-Confidence

Exercising reduces the risk of falling, increases your independence, and boosts your self-esteem, which makes you comfortable in social situations. When you can move around without worrying about falling and perform daily tasks without assistance, you will feel good about yourself and your life.

Regular exercise improves your well-being and health. It also encourages socialization, which boosts your mood. These factors contribute to increasing your confidence. High self-esteem and a positive attitude encourage older adults to continue exercising and leading a healthy lifestyle.

Physical activities build your self-esteem in a number of ways.

Boosts Your Energy

Your energy declines with age, which affects your mood and causes constant fatigue. It can be hard to start exercising when you are tired, but when you do, it can boost your energy.

High energy levels will increase your confidence because you will be active and able to take care of your needs. The more you exercise, the more energy you will have and the higher your self-esteem will be.

Gets You in Shape

When you look good, you feel good. Regular exercise and a healthy diet keep you in shape and help you maintain your weight, which will boost your self-esteem.

Provides a Sense of Accomplishment

Sticking to a workout routine and reaping its benefits can give you a sense of accomplishment. You are able to overcome any physical challenge and lead an active and healthy lifestyle. Achieving one's goals can have a huge impact on one's self-esteem.

Makes You Feel Empowered

Exercising increases your strength, giving you the ability to go to the grocery store, cook, and take care of all your other needs. Feeling healthy, strong, and capable is empowering and can increase your confidence.

Improves Your Mood

Regular exercise elevates your mood and reduces your stress. People who have a positive attitude usually feel good about themselves. Your mood and self-esteem are connected – when one is high, it lifts the other.

28-Day Program

This part provides a 28-day plan that addresses different parts of the body and muscles with rest days so you can take a break and allow your muscles to heal.

Day 1: Seated Backbend

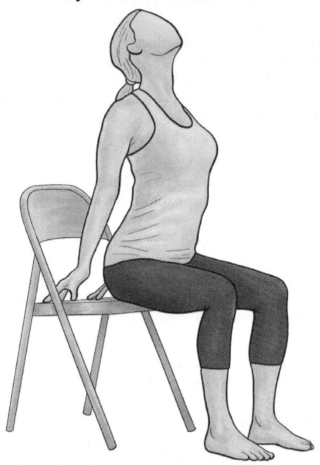

Seated Backbend.

Instructions:

1. Sit tall in a chair.
2. Keep your feet planted on the ground.
3. Place your hands on your thighs or behind your back, like in the video.
4. Take a long, deep breath and lengthen your spine while engaging your core muscles.
5. Breathe out and slowly lean back.
6. Keep your chest lifted while gazing forward.

7. Continue leaning backward and allow your upper back to arch gently. Keep your lower back supported.
8. Be careful not to strain yourself and pause once you feel a stretch in your back.
9. Hold the position for 10 to 20 seconds.
10. Take another deep breath while maintaining an open posture and expanding your chest.
11. Breathe out and sit in an upright position.
12. Take a moment to feel the impact of the exercise on your back.
13. Repeat three times.

Day 2: Chair Push-Ups

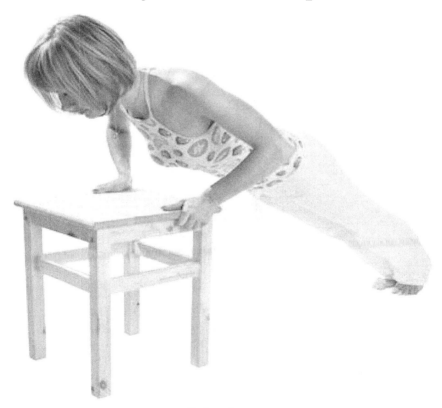

Chair push-ups.
Designed by Freepik. Source: https://www.freepik.com/free-photo/red-haired-girl-performing-fitness-exercises_12051 29.htm#fromView=search&page=1&position=21&uuid=8f489c21-918f-42f5-924f-802a0c21353b

Instructions:

1. Face your chair and put both hands on its sides.
2. Push your feet back to create a diagonal line with your body from your feet to your head.
3. Bend your elbows and slowly lower your chest toward the chair while keeping your body in a straight line.
4. Slowly and gently return to your starting position.
5. Repeat five to ten times.

Day 3: Tummy Twists

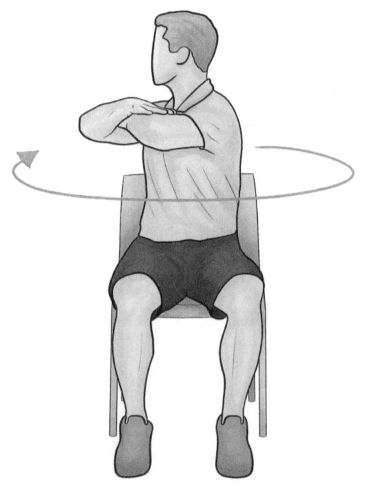

Tummy twists.

Instructions:

1. Sit in an upright position with your feet pressed firmly on the ground.
2. Put your right hand on your left arm and your left hand on your right arm, like in the video.
3. To activate your core muscles, breathe in and focus on stiffening your stomach muscles.
4. Twist your torso to the right, then return to the center.
5. Twist your torso to the left, then return to the center.
6. Repeat 10 times while alternating sides.

Day 4: Seated Jack

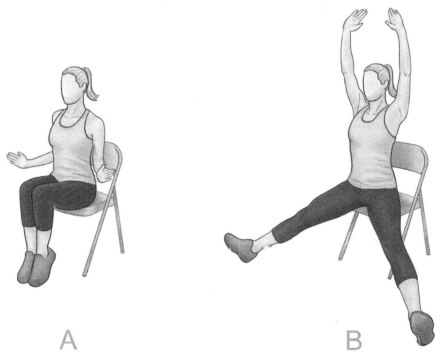

A   B

Seated Jacks.

Instructions:

1. Sit in an upright position with your torso away from the back of the chair.

2. Put your feet together and raise your arms to a right angle. Your upper arms should be parallel to the floor.

3. Close your arms together and push your feet out to the sides, similar to a jumping jack motion, while opening your arms to the sides.

4. Squeeze your shoulders together and return to your starting position.

5. Repeat ten times.

Day 5: Single-Arm Row

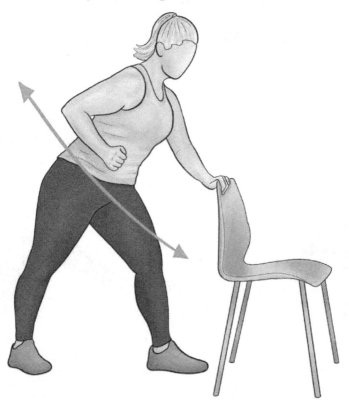

Single-Arm Row.

Instructions:

1. Stand next to your chair with your feet planted firmly on the ground.

2. Lean forward toward your chair and place one hand on the top of its back or on its seat (choose whatever feels comfortable).

3. Your back should be flat.
4. Pull your arm toward your chest, keeping your elbow close to your body.
5. Then, slowly extend your arm out.
6. Repeat ten times.

N.B. You can do this exercise with a dumbbell, but give yourself time to adapt to the routine before using weights.

Day 6: Meditation

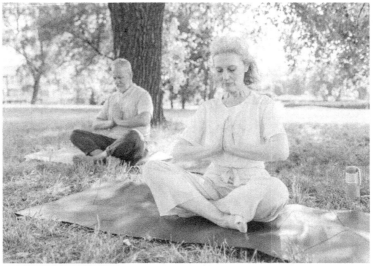

Meditation.

Exercising every day can be demanding for your body. You need to take breaks to give your muscles a chance to recover. You can take advantage of this time to rest your mind and body with meditation and breathing exercises.

Instructions:
1. Find a quiet room away from distractions.
2. Sit up straight in a comfortable position.
3. Take long and deep breaths.
4. Close your eyes and focus on your breathing.
5. Feel the air as it enters your body through your nostrils and flows through you.

6. Feel as it exits your body and takes with it all your stresses and worries.
7. Your mind may wander away, and distracting thoughts may creep in.
8. Don't focus on these thoughts – let them pass.
9. Bring your attention back to your breathing.
10. Stay in this calming state for 15 to 20 minutes.

Day 7: Breathing Exercise

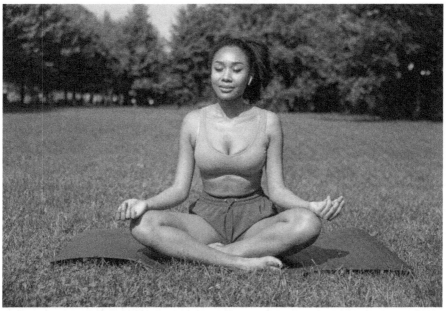

Breathing exercise.
https://www.pexels.com/photo/fit-ethnic-woman-practicing-yoga-in-park-5384531/

Instructions:

1. Sit on a chair and relax your head and body.
2. Take a deep breath through your nose while keeping your mouth closed.
3. Count to two.
4. Purse your lips as if you are whistling.
5. Breathe out through your lips while counting to four.
6. Repeat ten times.

Day 8: Kick Back

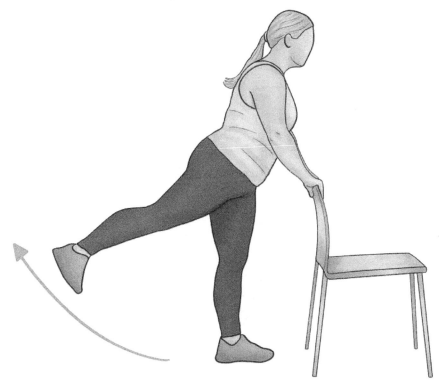

Kick back.

Instructions:

1. Stand and face the back of your chair while keeping your feet 12 inches away from it.

2. Put both hands on the top of the chair's back.

3. Engage the glute muscles and extend your left leg behind you. Point your toes down.

4. Hold this position for ten seconds. You should feel a contraction in the glute muscles.

5. Lower your left leg and return to your starting position.

6. Repeat five times, then switch to your right leg.

7. Keep your movements slow and controlled.

Day 9: Shoulder Circles

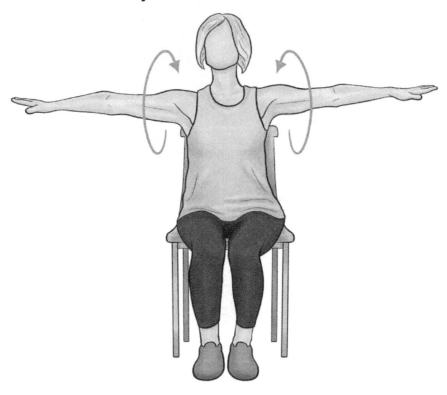

Shoulder circles.

Instructions:

1. With your feet planted firmly on the ground and your chest up, put both arms on your side.

2. Slowly and with controlled movements, move your shoulders forward in a circular motion. Lift them up and around, then return to the original position.

3. Repeat ten times, then switch to backward motion and repeat ten times.

Day 10: Heel Slides

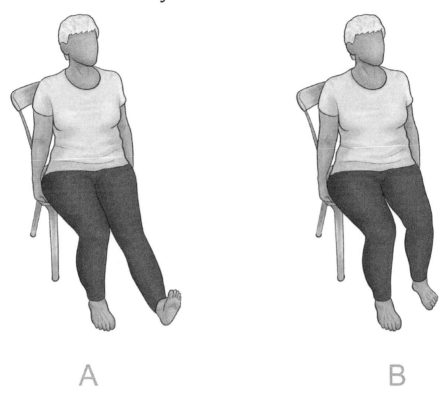

Heel Slides

Instructions:

1. Sit on the edge of your chair.

2. Extend your right leg out until it's straight, with your toes facing the ceiling and your heel on the ground.

3. Your left foot should be planted firmly on the ground at a 90-degree angle.

4. Slide your right heel very close to the chair with your right foot on the floor.

5. Repeat ten times, then switch foot.

Day 11: Knees to Chest

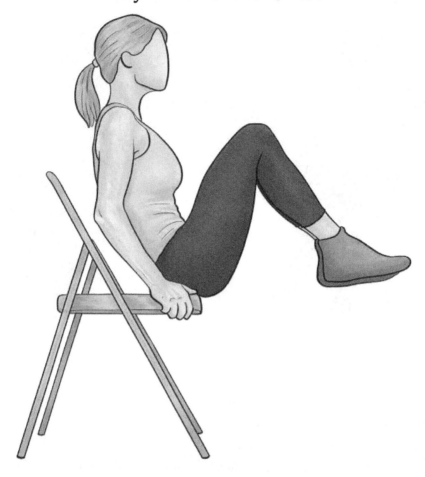

Knees to chest.

Instructions:

1. Sit on your chair and lean back slightly.
2. Hold the sides with both hands.
3. Take a long and deep breath to activate your core.
4. Lift your legs off the ground and extend them outward (your toes should point to the ceiling).
5. Bend your knees and bring them to your chest.
6. Pause, then reverse the motion.
7. Repeat ten times.

Day 12: Leg Extensions

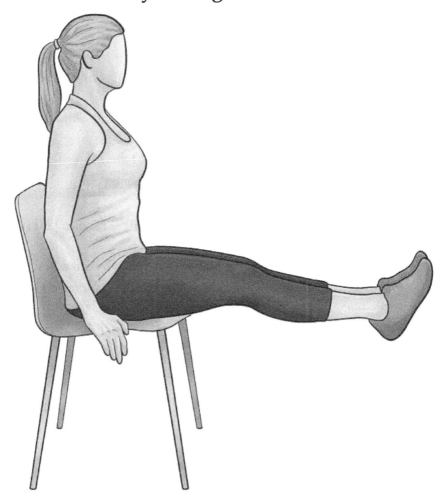

Leg Extensions.

Instructions:

1. Sit on the chair's edge and hold the chair with both hands.
2. Lean back slightly and extend your legs outward (your toes should face the ceiling, and your heels should touch the ground).
3. Engage the core and lift your legs toward the ceiling (you can practice with both legs or with one at a time).
4. Hold the position for a few seconds, then lower your legs.
5. Repeat 10 times.

Day 13: Meditation

You have finished your second week of exercises; it's time for some relaxation.

Instructions:

1. Lie on your back in a relaxing position with your arms by your side and your eyes closed.
2. Take a few deep breaths and clear your mind until you feel relaxed.
3. Focus on your toes and the sensation behind them.
4. Imagine each breath you take is flowing through your toes.
5. Remain in this state for five seconds.
6. Move your focus to your soles and notice any sensation you might be feeling.
7. Imagine the air you are breathing flowing through your soles.
8. Then, move to your calves, knees, thighs, hips, torso, abdomen, upper back, chest, shoulders, neck, and head to scan your entire body.
9. Notice if there is discomfort in any part of your body.
10. After you finish, relax for a couple of minutes in silence.
11. Then, open your eyes and stretch.

Day 14: Breathing Exercise

Instructions:

1. Sit up straight in a comfortable position.
2. Put your right hand on your chest and your left hand on your stomach.
3. Take a long and deep breath through your nostrils.
4. Feel your stomach rising and your chest moving a little.
5. Breathe out through your mouth and release all the air in your body while contracting your abdominal muscles.
6. Feel your stomach move as you breathe out.
7. Repeat 10 times.

Day 15: Squat to Chair

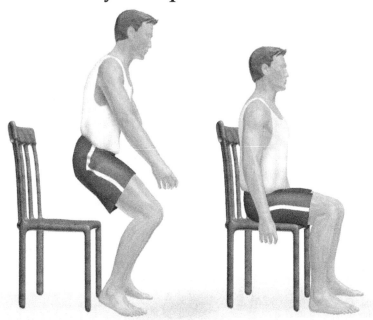

Chair Squat

Chair squat.

Instructions:

1. Stand upright with your back close to the front of the chair.
2. Keep your feet shoulder-width apart and put your chest up with your toes pointing outward.
3. Engage your core and start squatting down toward the chair.
4. Only touch the seat with your glutes; don't sit.
5. Push into your feet and return to your original position.
6. Repeat ten times.

Day 16: Modified Burpees

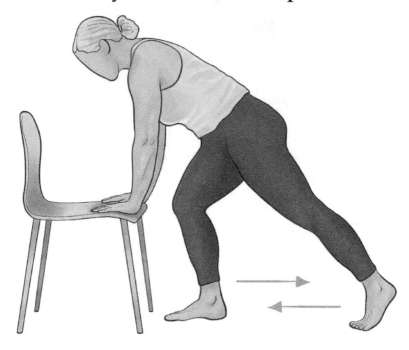

Modified Burpees.

Instructions:

1. Place a chair against the wall.
2. The back of the chair should be against the wall, and the seat should face you. To prevent accidents, make sure the chair isn't sliding or moving.
3. Stand facing the chair with your feet about a shoulder apart.
4. Press your hips back and bend your knees as if you are squatting.
5. Extend your arms and place your hands on the chair's seat. Your palms should be aligned.
6. Place your left foot behind the right one. Take a plank position.
7. Reverse the movement and put each foot forward to return to the starting position.
8. Extend your hips and knees while pressing through your feet to stand and lift your arms.
9. Repeat six to ten times.

Day 17: Ankle and Wrist Rolls

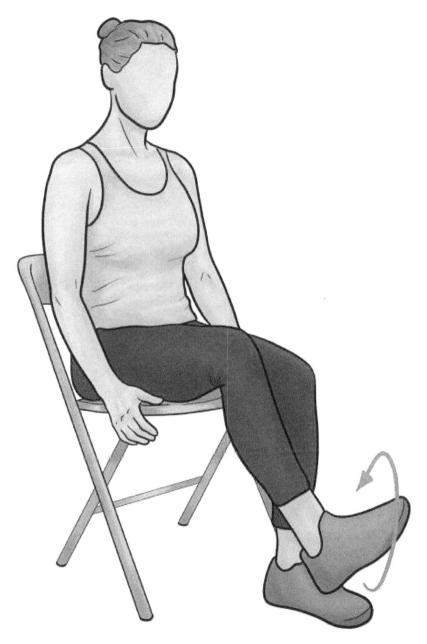

Ankle rolls.

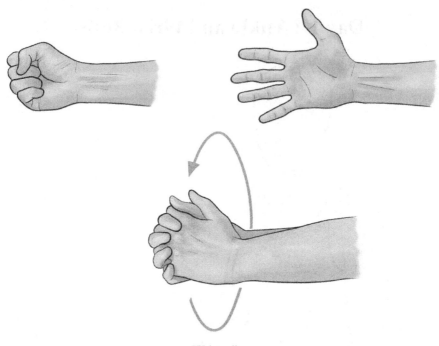

Wrist rolls.

Instructions:

1. Sit up straight in a chair.
2. Open and close your fists a few times to flex your fingers.
3. Put your hands together and roll your wrists ten times.
4. After you finish, flex your feet by curling and straightening your toes.
5. Roll your right ankle ten times, then your left ankle.

Day 18: Arm Raises

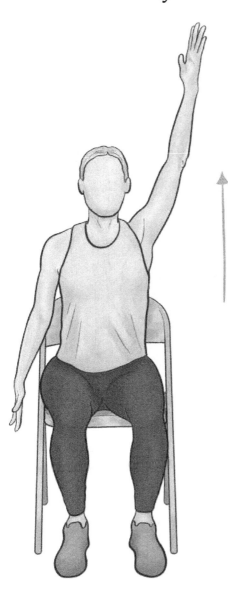

Instructions:

1. Sit in an upright position, with both arms on your side and both feet planted firmly on the ground.

2. Raise your left arm over your head without moving your body. Keep it straight.

3. Hold this position for three seconds.

4. Return to your starting position, then repeat with your right arm.

5. Repeat ten times for each arm.

Arm raises.

Day 19: Back Straightening and Stretching

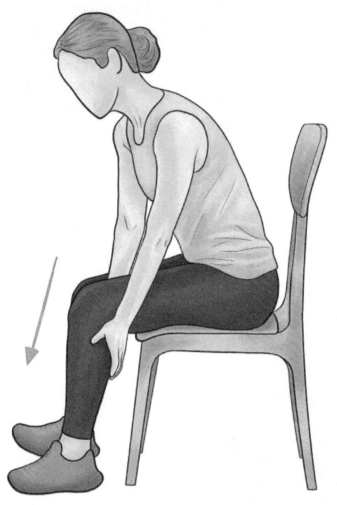

Back Straightening and Stretching.

Instructions:

1. Sit on your chair and keep both legs shoulder-length apart.
2. Put both hands under your left knee.
3. Slide your hands slowly from your knee to your ankle.
4. Hold this position for three seconds.
5. Switch sides and repeat.
6. Repeat ten times.

Day 20: Visualization

Instructions:

1. Sit or lie down and get comfortable.
2. Close your eyes and imagine you are in a relaxing and beautiful place.
3. Keep your imagination as vivid as possible.
4. Feel, taste, smell, hear, and see everything around you in the world you have created (for example, if you are on a beach, see the sun shining bright in the sky, hear the birds chirping, smell the trees, feel the water on your feet, and taste the fresh air.)
5. Let all your stresses go, and spend your time exploring the place.
6. After you finish, slowly open your eyes.

Day 21: Breathing Exercise

Instructions:

1. Sit in a comfortable position and close your eyes.
2. Relax your body and face.
3. Place a finger from each hand on your tragus to cover your ears.
4. Breathe in and gently press your fingers into the cartilage as you breathe out, keeping your mouth closed.
5. Make a humming noise like a bee.
6. Repeat ten times.

Day 22: Heel-to-Toe Raise

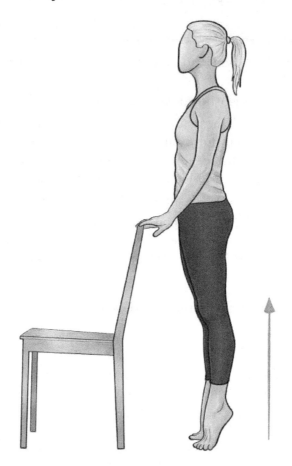

Heel-to-Toe Raise

Instructions:

1. Stand up straight next to your chair.
2. Keep your feet shoulder-width apart.
3. Hold the back of the chair with both hands.
4. Stand on your toes while holding the chair for support.
5. Stay in this position for two seconds.
6. Return to the starting position.
7. Raise your toes while your ankles are still on the floor.
8. Repeat ten times.

Day 23: Hip Extension

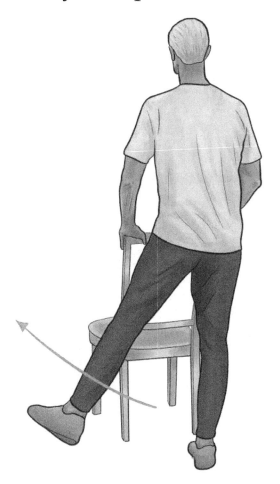

Hip extension.

Instructions:

1. Stand behind your chair.
2. Hold onto its back with both hands for support.
3. Slowly and gently raise your right leg behind you. Don't bend your waist.
4. Return to the starting position.
5. Repeat ten times, then switch legs and repeat for another ten times.

Day 24: Skater Switch

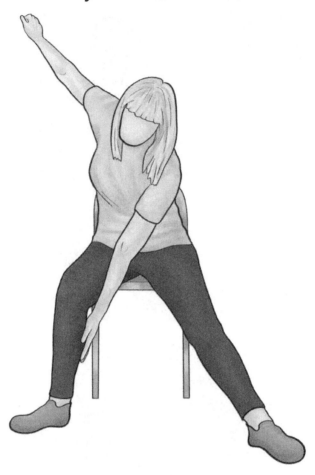

Skater switch.

Instructions:

1. Sit on the edge of your chair and bend your left knee with your left toe on the ground.
2. Stretch your right leg out to the side.
3. Bend forward and stretch your arms out in front of you.
4. Lift your left arm behind your body and bend it at the waist.
5. Reach your right arm to the bottom of your left foot.
6. Sit in an upright position and bring your arms forward.
7. Repeat ten times, then switch foot.

Day 25: Touch the Floor

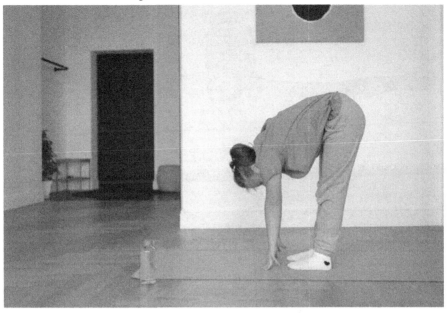

Touch the floor.

Designed by Freepik. https://www.freepik.com/free-photo/girl-doing-yoga-poses-side-view_33809757.htm#fromView=search&page=1&position=3&uuid=6218994e-8626-4a25-a78f-8de7c0811623

Instructions:

1. Sit up straight with your feet planted firmly on the ground and roll back your shoulders.
2. Keep your legs shoulder-length apart to allow movement.
3. Lean forward and hinge from the waist while keeping your back straight.
4. Touch the floor with your fingertips.
5. Return to the first position and take a few deep breaths.
6. Repeat ten times.

Day 26: Seated Ts

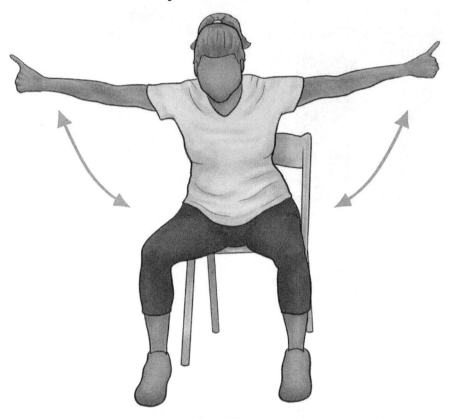

Seated Ts.

Instructions:

1. Sit on a chair with your feet shoulder-width apart.
2. Lean forward while keeping your back straight and extending your hands.
3. Raise your hands with your pinky finger sticking out.
4. When your arms reach shoulder level, bring them down.
5. Repeat ten times.

Day 27: Yoga Breathing Exercise

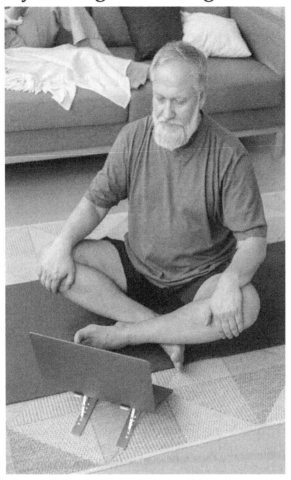

Yoga Breathing Exercise.
https://www.pexels.com/photo/man-person-people-relaxation-7529994/

Instructions:

1. Sit in a comfortable position.
2. Curl your tongue and stick it out (if you can't curl your tongue, purse your lips).
3. Take a long and deep breath through your mouth.
4. Breathe out through your nostrils.
5. Repeat for five minutes.

Day 28: Breathing Exercise

Instructions:

1. Take a long, deep breath through your nostrils while counting to five.

2. Breathe out through your nose while counting to five.

3. Repeat for ten minutes.

How to Integrate Exercise Routines into Your Daily Life

- Exercise first thing in the morning, right after you wake up, and before you start your day. Set your alarm 10 or 15 minutes early so you can exercise alone and in peace.

- Make time for exercising every day and schedule it in your calendar. Treat it as a priority and schedule everything else in your day around it.

- Exercise with a friend or a family member to motivate each other.

- Choose exercises that you enjoy and stay away from ones that make you uncomfortable.

- Exercise at home, outdoors, or while watching TV to avoid boredom.

Consistency is key. Your exercise routine should be an essential part of your daily life – as should be sleeping and eating. Prioritize it and give it a few minutes every day. Consider it an investment in your health. When you are consistent in your routine, it becomes a part of your lifestyle.

Practice chair exercises every day and allow yourself two days to relax your mind and body. During this time, take care of your mental health and practice meditation and breathing exercises.

Chapter 3: Upper-Body Strength

Aging is a natural process that should be embraced with grace. During this time, keeping yourself physically active becomes necessary for maintaining health. For seniors like yourself, focusing on upper-body strength and mobility is the key, and chair exercises for upper-body strength can be a practical and safe solution. These seated workouts are designed to be gentle yet effective, keeping in mind the mobility challenges many face.

Chair exercises for the upper body specifically target essential muscle groups in your arms, shoulders, chest, and back. Besides improved upper-body strength, you will have increased joint mobility and flexibility. The stability provided by the chair during these exercises greatly improves balance, significantly reducing the risk of falls.

It's the accessibility and convenience of chair exercises that allow you to perform them almost anywhere. All you need is a sturdy chair and knowing the right moves to execute. Whether you aim to maintain independence, seek engaging activities, or look for low-impact options, keep reading for specific chair exercises tailored for you. It can be another addition to your journey toward enhanced well-being.

Daily Activities and Upper-Body Strength

Here are some daily activities where your upper-body strength becomes a vital force:

Reaching and Grasping

The seemingly mundane task of reaching for items on high shelves or grasping objects in your daily activities requires upper-body strength. These movements are intricately linked to the strength of your arms and shoulders. Your upper-body strength ensures that these motions are executed effortlessly, preventing any strain or discomfort in your day-to-day tasks.

Dressing Independence

Dressing up involves several upper-body movements, from reaching overhead to put on a shirt to reaching behind when wearing a blazer.

Carrying and Lifting

When carrying groceries or lifting a bag, your arms and shoulders bear the load in numerous daily tasks.

Reducing Reliance on Assistance

A decline in your upper-body strength could potentially lead to an increased reliance on other muscles for assistance in daily activities.

Promoting Postural Stability

Your upper-body strength is also necessary for maintaining an upright and stable posture. This balance prevents falls, substantially reducing the risk of accidents and enhancing your overall safety.

Incorporating targeted exercises that focus on strengthening your upper body can make a positive change. Chair exercises designed for your upper body can be a foundation for maintaining and enhancing your strength, actively contributing to your well-being.

Furthermore, please remember that preserving your upper-body strength is not a mere fitness goal; it is an essential component of a lifestyle that actively promotes continued independence and a higher level of functionality in your daily activities.

Exercises for Upper-Body Strength
Seated Arm Raises

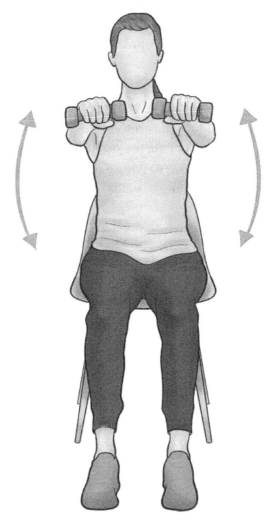

Seated arm raises.

Instructions:

1. Sit at the edge of the chair, ensuring your back is straight and your feet are flat on the floor.

2. Hold a weight in each hand, palms facing your thighs.

3. Keep your shoulders relaxed.

Movement:

4. Inhale slowly and lift both arms straight in front of you.

5. Maintain a slight bend in your elbows throughout the movement.

6. Reach toward shoulder height, feeling the engagement in your shoulders and upper arms.

7. Exhale and slowly lower your arms back down to your thighs, controlling the descent.

Variation:

- For added resistance, consider using heavier weights.

- If you have shoulder concerns or are new to exercising, lift one arm at a time while keeping the opposite hand on your thigh.

- Remember never to use weights that are too heavy, as it can lead to shoulder strain or muscle injury.

Seated Shoulder Press

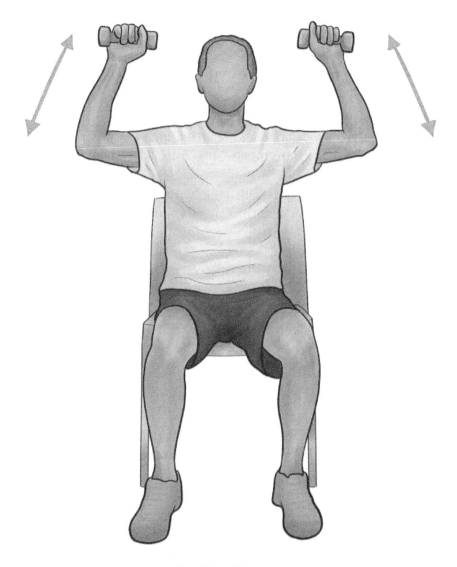

Seated shoulder press.

Instructions:

1. Sit comfortably with a straight back, holding a weight in each hand at shoulder height and your palms facing forward.
2. Ensure your feet are flat on the floor.

Movement:

3. Inhale deeply and press the weights overhead, extending your arms without locking your elbows.

4. Feel the contraction in your shoulder muscles at the top of the movement.

5. Exhale slowly and lower the weights back down to shoulder height while maintaining control.

Variation:

- If you are a beginner and want to increase your control over these exercise movements, use resistance bands instead of weights.

- If you have concerns with your wrists, perform the movement without weights or resistance bands and focus on the controlled motion.

Seated Chest Squeeze

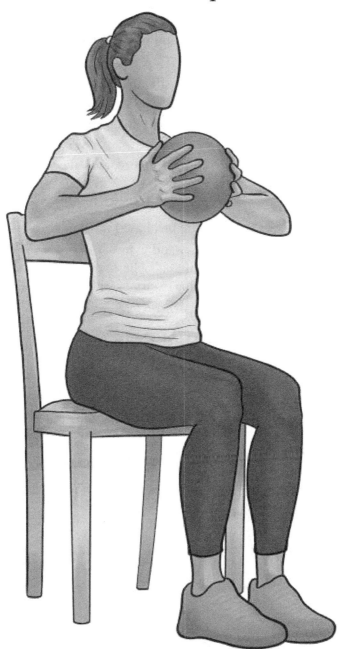

Seated chest squeeze.

Instructions:

1. Sit with an upright posture, holding a softball or cushion at chest level with both hands.

2. Ensure your back is straight and your shoulders are relaxed.

Movement:

3. Inhale deeply and squeeze the ball or cushion between your hands, engaging your chest muscles.

4. Focus on bringing your shoulder blades together without leaning forward.

5. Exhale slowly and release the squeeze, allowing your chest muscles to relax.

Variation:

• Adjust the pressure on the ball based on your comfort level.

• People with arthritis or hand issues can use a softer ball for reduced resistance. Still, it's best to consult a healthcare professional, as performing exercises with a pre-existing condition can elevate the issue.

Seated Row

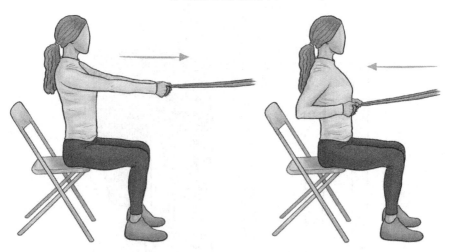

Seated row.

Instructions:

1. Sit tall at the edge of the chair, holding onto resistance bands or weights with your arms extended in front of you.

2. Ensure your back is in an upright position and your feet are flat on the floor.

Movement:

3. Inhale deeply and pull your elbows back, squeezing your shoulder blades together.
4. Keep your wrists straight and close to your body during the entire movement.
5. Exhale slowly and release, extending your arms back to the starting position with control.

Variation:

- Adjust resistance band tension based on your strength level.
- For those with back concerns, sit against a backrest for additional support.

Seated Twist

Seated Twist.

Instructions:

1. Sit with a straight back, holding a lightweight or a physio ball with both hands at chest level.
2. Keep your feet grounded to the floor.

Movement:

3. Exhale slowly and twist your torso to one side, allowing your head to follow the movement.
4. Inhale deeply and return to the center, maintaining good posture.
5. Repeat the twist on the other side, feeling a gentle stretch in your torso.

Variation:

- Gradually increase the weight for added challenge.
- For people with back issues, perform a gentler twist, focusing on mobility rather than intensity. Deep waist twisting and bending are not recommended for people suffering from lumbar arthritis.

Seated Bicep Curls

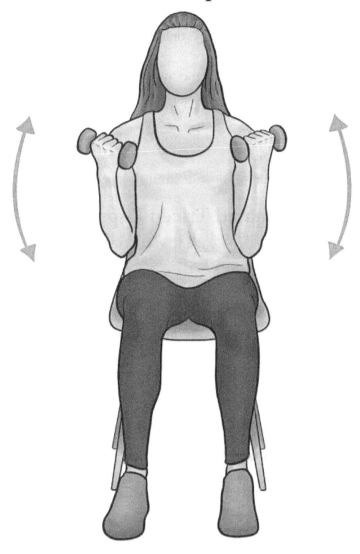

Seated bicep curls.

Instructions:

1. Sit with your back straight, holding a weight in each hand and your palms facing forward.

2. Keep your elbows close to your body and your feet flat on the floor.

Movement:

3. Inhale deeply and curl the weights toward your shoulders, contracting your biceps.

4. Maintain a controlled and deliberate movement, focusing on muscle engagement.

5. Exhale slowly and lower the weights back down, keeping the movement smooth.

Variation:

- For a variation, perform hammer curls by keeping your palms facing each other.

- Adjust the weight to suit your strength level.

Seated Tricep Dips

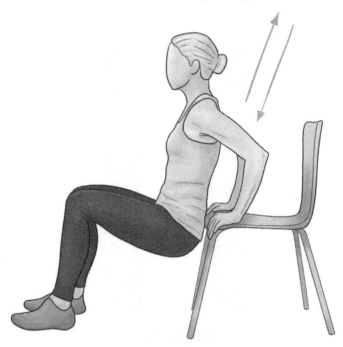

Seated Tricep Dips.

Instructions:

1. Sit at the edge of the chair with your hands gripping the front edge.

2. Slide your bottom off the chair, ensuring your feet are flat on the floor and your knees are bent.

Movement:

3. Inhale deeply and bend your elbows, lowering your body toward the floor.
4. Keep your back close to the chair and your elbows pointing straight back.
5. Exhale slowly and push through your palms, straightening your arms back to the starting position.

Variation:

- Adjust the distance of your feet from the chair to control difficulty.
- Focus on engaging your triceps throughout the movement.

Seated Leg Lifts

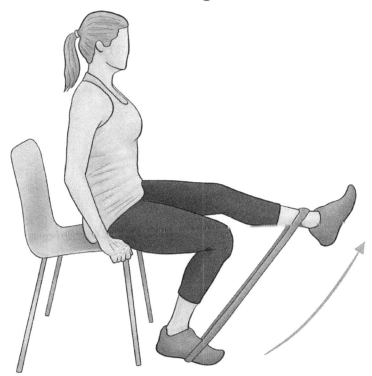

Seated leg lifts.

Instructions:

1. Sit tall with your back straight and your feet flat on the floor.
2. For support, grip the chair's sides.

Movement:

3. Inhale deeply and lift one leg straight in front of you, engaging your core.

4. Hold the lifted position for a few seconds, feeling the contraction in your quadriceps.

5. Exhale slowly and lower the leg back down, maintaining control.

Variation:

- For added challenges, incorporate ankle weights or resistance bands.

- Ensure proper stability by holding onto the chair or placing your hands on your hips.

- People suffering from back problems should consult a physiotherapist before engaging in this exercise, as it will impact the lumbar area (lower back).

Seated Side Leg Raises

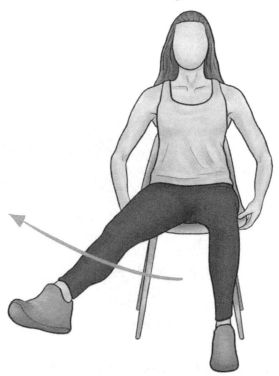

Seated leg raises.

Instructions:

1. Sit tall with your feet flat on the floor and your hands resting on your lap.
2. Engage your core for stability.

Movement:

3. Inhale deeply and lift one leg out to the side, keeping it straight.
4. Hold the lifted position for a moment, feeling the pressure in your outer thigh.
5. Exhale slowly and lower the leg back down to the starting position.

Variation:

- Adjust the height of the leg lift based on your comfort level.
- Focus on maintaining good posture and avoid leaning to the opposite side.

Seated Knee Extensions

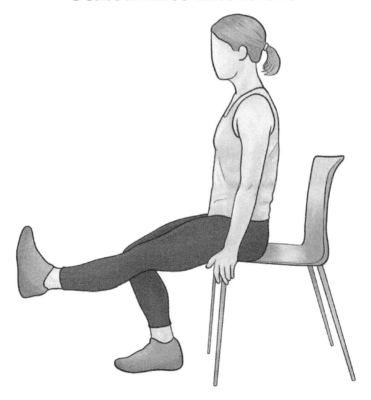

Seated knee extensions

Instructions:

1. Sit tall with your back straight and your feet flat on the floor.
2. For support, grip the chair's sides.

Movement:

3. Inhale deeply and extend one leg straight out in front of you, lifting the foot a few inches off the ground.
4. Engage your quadriceps and hold the extended position for a moment.
5. Exhale slowly and lower the leg back down, maintaining control.

Variation:

- Increase difficulty by placing a small weight on the ankle.
- Ensure stability by holding onto the chair or placing your hands on your hips.

Seated Heel Taps

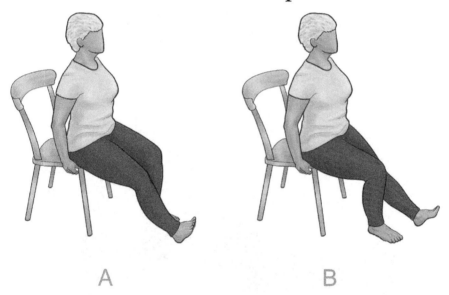

A   B

Seated heel taps.

Instructions:

1. Sit with your back straight and your feet flat on the floor.
2. Hold onto the sides of the chair for stability.

Movement:

3. Inhale deeply and lift one foot slightly off the floor.
4. Tap your heel on the ground, alternating between each foot.
5. Keep the movement controlled and rhythmic.

Variation:

• Increase the speed for a cardiovascular element.

• Focus on maintaining stability and controlled tapping motions.

Seated Marching

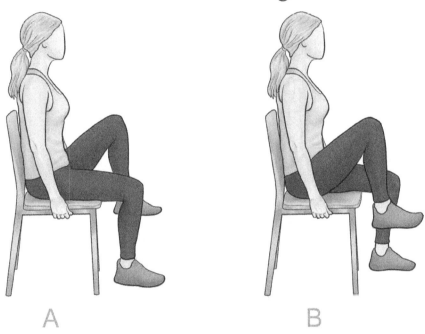

A   B

Seated marching.

Instructions:

1. Sit tall with your back straight and your feet flat on the floor.
2. For support, grip the chair's sides.

Movement:

3. Inhale deeply and lift one knee toward your chest.
4. Lower the lifted leg while simultaneously lifting the other knee in a marching motion.

5. Continue alternating between each leg in a controlled and rhythmic manner.

Variation:

- Lift your knees higher for added intensity.
- Focus on engaging your core and maintaining stability throughout the movement.

Seated Torso Stretch

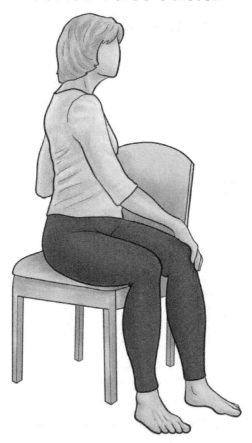

Seated torso stretch.

Instructions:

1. Sit tall with your feet flat on the floor.
2. Place one hand on the opposite knee, ensuring your back is straight.

Movement:

3. Inhale deeply and twist your torso to one side, using your hand on the knee to guide the movement.
4. Hold the stretch for 15 to 30 seconds, feeling a gentle rotation in your spine.
5. Exhale slowly and return to the center.
6. Repeat the stretch on the other side.

Variation:

- Adjust the intensity of the stretch by either twisting further or less.
- Ensure your back remains straight and the movement is controlled.

Seated High Knees

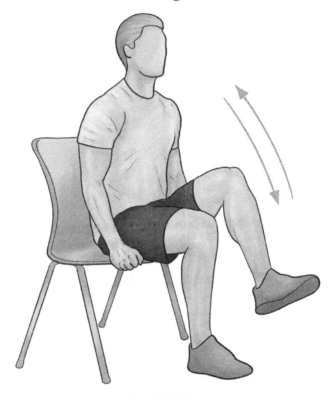

Seated high knees.

Instructions:

1. Sit with your back straight and your feet flat on the floor.

2. Hold onto the sides of the chair for stability.

Movement:

3. Inhale deeply and lift one knee toward your chest.
4. Quickly switch to the other knee, creating a marching motion with a higher knee lift.
5. Continue alternating between each knee in a controlled and rhythmic manner.

Variation:

- Increase the speed for a higher cardiovascular impact.
- Focus on maintaining stability and controlled high-knee movements.

Seated Ankle Rolls

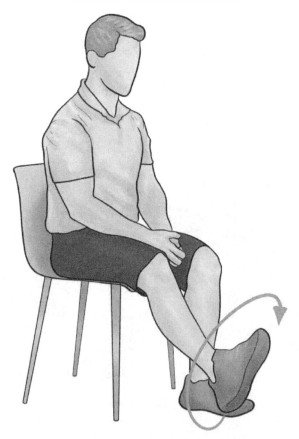

Seated ankle rolls.

Instructions:

1. Sit tall with your feet flat on the floor.
2. Lift one foot and rotate your ankle in a circular motion.

Movement:

3. Inhale deeply and perform ankle rolls in a clockwise direction.
4. Feel the stretch and movement in your ankle joint.
5. Exhale slowly and switch to counterclockwise ankle rolls.
6. Perform the movement in both directions for each ankle.

Variation:

- Adjust the size of the ankle circles based on your comfort level.
- Ensure a smooth and controlled motion throughout the ankle rolls.

Integrating these chair exercises into your regular fitness routine can significantly boost your well-being. Here's a concise roadmap for incorporating these exercises into a balanced and effective program:

Warm-up

You can start with a gentle warm-up to increase blood flow and prepare the body for exercise. Consider incorporating seated marching, ankle rolls, and torso stretches. Perform each movement for 5 to 10 minutes to gradually elevate the heart rate and loosen up the joints. In addition to these exercises, you can do any warm-up exercise you want.

Strength Training

As part of your strength-training routine, include chair exercises that target the upper body, like seated arm raises, seated shoulder presses, seated chest squeezes, seated rows, and seated bicep curls. Aim for 2 to 3 sets of 10 to 15 repetitions for each exercise. Adjust the weight or resistance to challenge yourself without compromising your control.

Cardiovascular Exercise

You should consider adding seated exercises involving dynamic movements, like seated high knees and seated marching, in order to improve your cardiovascular health. Perform these exercises at moderate intensity for 15 to 30 minutes to enhance heart health and endurance.

Flexibility and Mobility

Include seated stretches like the seated torso stretch to improve flexibility and maintain joint health. At the end of your routine, perform static stretches, holding each stretch for 15 to 30 seconds. Remember to stay focused on major muscle groups, including shoulders, chest, and legs.

Balance and Stability

Add seated leg lifts, side leg raises, and knee extensions to enhance balance and stability during movement. Besides engaging the leg muscles, these exercises also engage the core muscles of the back to improve control. Include them 2 to 3 times a week, aiming for 2 to 3 sets of 10 to 15 repetitions for each leg-related exercise.

Cool Down

Finish your routine with a cool-down to lower your heart rate and promote relaxation. Perform gentle seated stretches, such as the seated ankle rolls and seated knee extensions, to ease tension and prevent muscle stiffness.

Frequency and Progression

Start with two to three sessions per week, gradually increasing the frequency as your fitness level improves. As you become more comfortable with the exercises, consider progressing by increasing the number of sets, repetitions, or resistance. Listen to your body, and if you experience any discomfort, either adjust the intensity or consult with a fitness professional.

Rest Days

Incorporate rest days into your routine to allow your body time to recover. On these days, focus on light activities like walking or gentle stretching to promote circulation and flexibility.

Consultation with a Healthcare Provider

Before starting any new fitness routine, especially for seniors or for individuals with pre-existing health conditions, consult with your healthcare provider. They can provide personalized guidance based on your health status and ensure the exercises are safe and suitable for you.

Long-Term Benefits

Maintaining upper-body strength through regular exercise yields a multitude of long-term benefits that contribute to well-being and independence. Here are some key advantages:

Enhanced Functional Independence

Now, you already know that improved upper-body strength enables better performance of daily activities like lifting groceries, reaching for objects, and maintaining good posture. The ability to independently perform routine tasks enhances overall quality of life and improves self-reliance.

Reduced Risk of Falls

A strong upper body supports better balance and stability, reducing the risk of falls, which is crucial for anyone who may be prone to accidents.

Joint Health and Flexibility

Strengthening the muscles surrounding the shoulders, arms, and upper back supports the joints, reducing the risk of joint-related issues. You will be improving flexibility with these exercises, aiding in the maintenance of a full range of motion.

Bone Health

Weight-bearing exercises for the upper body, especially those involving resistance, contribute to bone density, reducing the risk of osteoporosis.

Pain Management

Strengthening the upper back and shoulders promotes better posture, which can alleviate chronic pain associated with poor alignment. Strong upper-body muscles can reduce tension in the neck and shoulders, easing discomfort and improving overall comfort.

Cardiovascular Health

Engaging in exercises that elevate the heart rate, like seated marching or high knees, improves cardiovascular health, reducing the risk of heart-related issues.

Mood and Mental Health

Exercise, including upper-body strength training, triggers the release of endorphins, promoting a positive mood and reducing the risk of depression and anxiety. Regular physical activity has been linked to cognitive benefits, contributing to long-term brain health.

Weight Management

Caloric Expenditure: Strength training, even for the upper body, contributes to increased muscle mass, which, in turn, enhances metabolism and supports weight management.

Social Engagement

Group Activities: Participating in group exercise classes or community fitness programs can foster social connections, reduce feelings of isolation, and promote mental well-being.

Longevity and Vitality

Healthy Aging: Maintaining upper-body strength is a key component of healthy aging, allowing individuals to lead active and fulfilling lives well into their later years.

Adaptability to Aging Changes

Maintaining Function: As the body naturally undergoes age-related changes, having a strong upper body aids in adapting to these changes, ensuring continued functionality and independence.

The long-term benefits of maintaining upper-body strength extend beyond physical fitness. They encompass mental well-being, social engagement, and the ability to adapt to the challenges of aging, ultimately contributing to a healthier and more fulfilling life. Regular exercise, combined with a balanced lifestyle, is a powerful tool for promoting overall longevity and vitality.

Chapter 4: Lower-Body Empowerment

Lower-body exercises are crucial for seniors as they significantly contribute to overall health and independence. Muscle mass tends to decline as individuals age, decreasing strength and stability. Lower-body exercises, such as squats, lunges, and leg presses, help counteract this muscle loss, enhancing balance and preventing falls. Additionally, these exercises improve joint flexibility and bone density, reducing the risk of fractures and osteoporosis. Lower-body workouts also promote better circulation, aiding cardiovascular health. Incorporating lower-body exercises into a senior fitness routine fosters physical well-being, supports daily activities, and preserves a sense of autonomy.

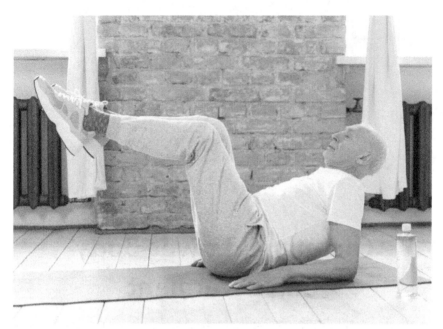

Lower-body exercises are crucial for seniors as they significantly contribute to overall health and independence.
Designed by Freepik. https://www.freepik.com/free-photo/full-shot-senior-man-training-indoors_13402651.htm#fromView=search&page=2&position=32&uuid=ce13450b-07a5-4e44-a34f-2634a4970.54a

Lower-body exercises are particularly vital for seniors due to their pivotal role in maintaining stability and mobility. As individuals age, there is a natural decline in muscle mass and strength, especially in the lower extremities. Strengthening the lower body through exercises like squats and lunges helps improve balance, prevent falls, and enhance overall stability. Additionally, these exercises contribute to better joint flexibility, supporting smooth and controlled movements. By focusing on the lower body, seniors can foster the muscle strength needed for daily activities, such as walking and climbing stairs, thus promoting independence and preserving a high level of mobility. Prioritizing lower-body workouts is key to sustaining a healthy and active lifestyle in later years.

Lower-Body Chair Exercises

Chair Squats

1. Begin seated with your feet hip-width apart and flat on the floor.
2. Stand up by extending your hips and knees.
3. Lower yourself back down to the seated position with controlled movement.

Variation/Modification:

Hold the chair armrests while standing up and sitting down for added support. To intensify, try standing without using armrests or add a brief pause at the standing position.

Seated Leg Extensions

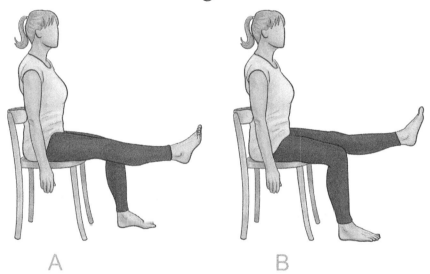

A   B

Seated leg extensions.

1. Sit tall with both feet flat on the floor.
2. Lift one leg straight out before you, then lower it back down.
3. Ensure a controlled motion and engage your core for stability.

Variation/Modification:

For increased difficulty, perform leg extensions simultaneously with both legs. Add ankle weights for extra resistance. If needed, use a chair with armrests for balance.

Chair Tap Dance

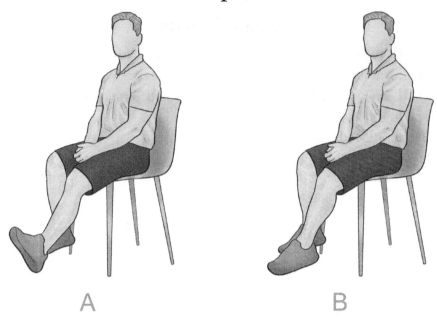

Chair tap dance

1. Sit comfortably with your back straight.
2. Tap your feet alternately on the ground, like a tapping dance.
3. Gradually increase the pace for a more dynamic workout.

Variation/Modification:

Elevate your knees higher during taps to engage the core and increase difficulty. Perform the taps at a slower pace for reduced impact.

Seated Toe Taps

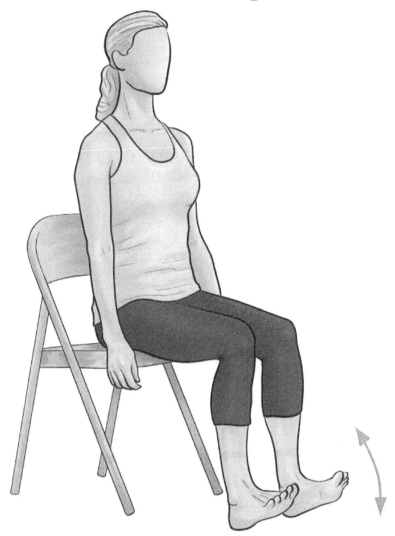

Seated toe taps.

1. Sit with your feet flat on the floor.
2. Tap your toes on the floor, lifting your heels slightly.
3. Gradually increase the speed of the toe taps.

Variation/Modification:

Lift your knees higher during toe taps to intensify the exercise. If necessary, perform at a slower pace for lower intensity.

Seated Side Leg Raises

1. Sit on the edge of the chair with your back straight.
2. Lift one leg to the side, then lower it back down with controlled movement.

Variation/Modification:

For an added challenge, use a resistance band around your thighs. Hold onto the chair for support if needed.

Seated Heel Raises

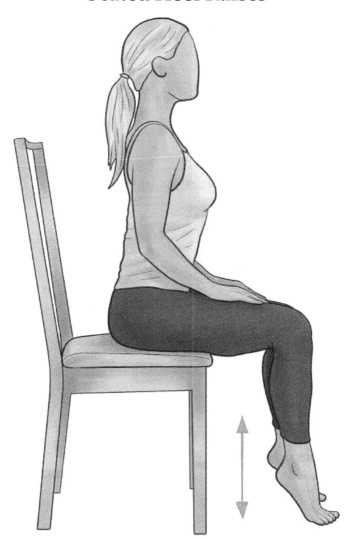

Seated heel raises.

1. Sit tall with your back straight.
2. Lift your heels off the ground, ensuring a controlled motion.
3. Lower your heels back down with control.

Variation/Modification:

Add ankle weights for increased resistance. Hold onto the chair for balance or perform seated heel raises one foot at a time for better stability.

Seated Leg Crosses

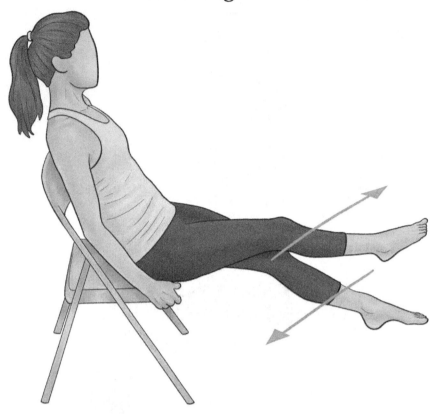

Seated leg crosses.

1. Sit tall with your back straight.
2. Cross one leg over the other at the ankles and then uncross them.
3. Alternate crossing and uncrossing your legs.

Variation/Modification:

Add a gentle twist in your upper body to engage the core further. For those needing less difficulty, perform the leg crosses slower.

Seated Torso Twist

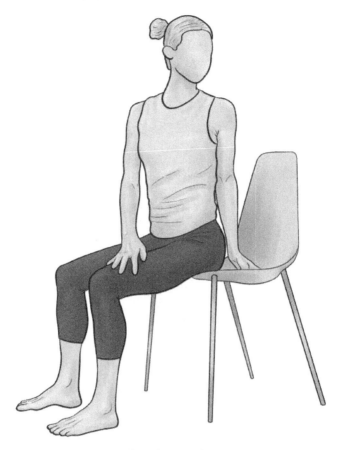

Seated torso twist.

1. Start in an upright, seated position at the edge of the chair, with your feet flat on the floor.

2. Engage your core and maintain a straight back.

3. Slowly rotate your torso to the right, bringing your right hand to the back of the chair and your left hand across your body.

4. Hold the twist for a moment, feeling a gentle stretch.

5. Return to the center and repeat the twist to the left.

Variation/Modification:

Hold a lightweight object with both hands during the twists to increase difficulty. For a gentler modification, perform the twists at a slower pace and with less range of motion.

Seated Arm Circles

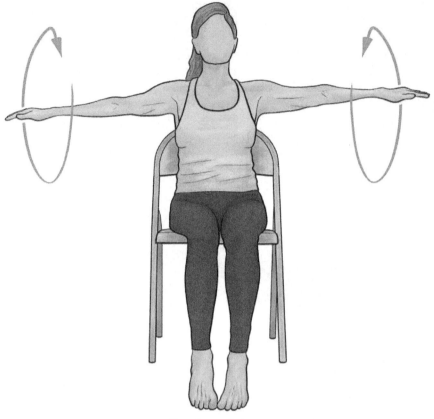

Seated arm circles.

1. Sit tall with your arms extended to the sides and your palms facing down.

2. Initiate small circular motions with your arms, first clockwise and then counterclockwise.

3. Ensure a controlled and deliberate movement, focusing on engaging the shoulder muscles.

4. Reverse the direction of the circles after completing one set.

Variation/Modification:

For added resistance, hold light weights in each hand. Adjust the size of the circles based on comfort and fitness level.

Seated Shoulder Shrugs

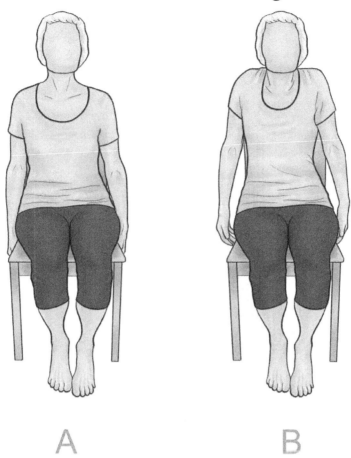

A   B

Seated shoulder shrugs.

1. Sit upright with your arms at your sides and your palms facing inward.

2. Elevate both shoulders toward your ears in a controlled manner.

3. Hold the shrug briefly, feeling the contraction in your shoulder muscles.

4. Lower your shoulders back down to the starting position.

Variation/Modification:

Intensify the exercise by holding lightweight objects or water bottles in each hand. Perform the shoulder shrugs at a slower pace for a gentler approach.

Seated Side Bends

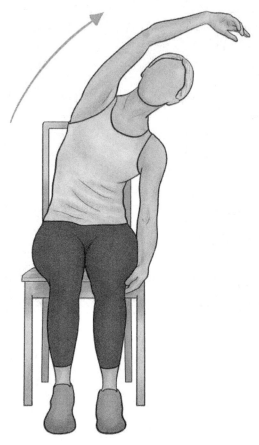

Seated side bends.

1. Sit with your feet flat, your back straight, and your hands on your hips.

2. Inhale and lean to the right, ensuring a smooth, controlled movement.

3. Hold the stretch for a moment, feeling the elongation along the left side of your torso.

4. Exhale and return to the upright position. Repeat the bend to the left.

Variation/Modification:

If needed, hold onto the chair for additional support. Adjust the range of motion based on your flexibility and comfort.

Seated Chest Press

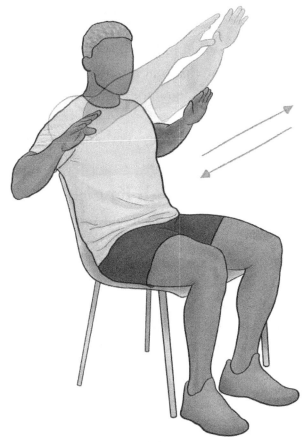

Seated chest press.

1. Sit on the edge of the chair with your feet flat and your back straight.
2. Extend both arms forward at shoulder height, palms facing each other.
3. Bring your arms back toward your chest, squeezing your pectoral muscles.
4. Ensure a controlled and deliberate movement throughout the exercise.

Variation/Modification:

Increase resistance by using resistance bands or holding light weights in each hand. Adjust the speed of the chest press to control the intensity.

Seated Tricep Dips

1. Sit at the edge of the chair, with your hands gripping the seat and your fingers pointing forward.
2. Lift your hips off the chair, moving them forward.
3. Bend your elbows, lowering your hips toward the ground.
4. Push through your palms to return to the starting position.

Variation/Modification:

Bend your knees to reduce difficulty. Perform tricep dips at a slower pace for a more controlled workout.

Seated High Knees

1. Sit upright with your back straight and your hands resting on the sides of the chair.
2. Lift your knees toward your chest alternately in a brisk manner.
3. Engage your core and maintain an upright posture.

Variation/Modification:

Hold onto the chair for balance and support. Increase the speed for a higher cardio workout or perform high knees at a slower pace for a milder exercise.

Seated Hip Flexor Stretch

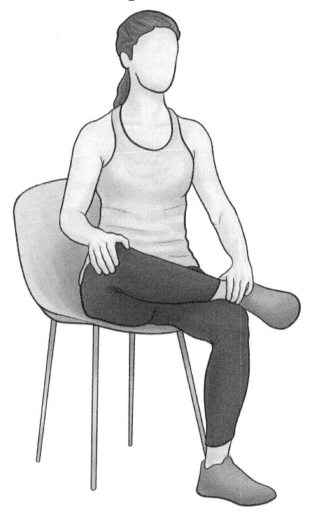

Seated hip flexor stretch.

1. Sit tall with your feet flat on the floor.
2. Cross your right ankle over your left knee.
3. Press down on the crossed knee, feeling a stretch in the right hip.
4. Hold the stretch, ensuring a comfortable and controlled position.

Variation/Modification:

Adjust the pressure based on comfort. Switch to stretching the left hip by crossing the left ankle over the right knee.

Seated Ankle Circles

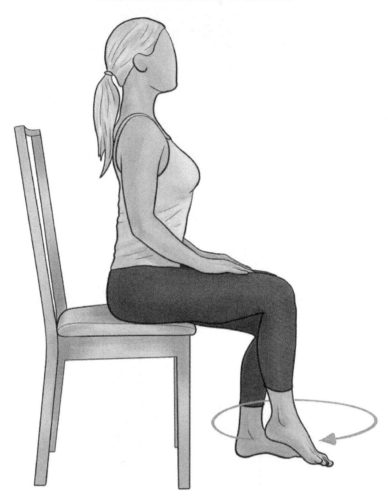

Seated ankle circles.

1. Lift one foot and rotate the ankle clockwise, then counterclockwise.

2. Switch to the other foot and repeat the ankle circles.

Variation/Modification:

Perform ankle circles in both directions. Depending on personal comfort, this exercise can be done in a seated or lying position.

Integrating Exercises in Your Routine

Integrating lower-body exercises into a routine is crucial for maintaining overall health, strength, and mobility. Whether you are a fitness enthusiast or just starting, incorporating lower-body exercises offers numerous benefits. Here's how you can effectively integrate them into your routine:

Balanced Workout Routine

Begin by creating a comprehensive workout plan covering various fitness aspects, including cardiovascular endurance, strength training, flexibility, and balance.

Allocate specific days for different types of exercises to ensure a balanced approach to overall fitness.

Frequency and Consistency

Aim for a consistent lower-body workout frequency, ideally incorporating lower-body exercises into your routine two to three times per week.

Consistency is crucial for seeing progress, so maintain a regular schedule.

Variety of Exercises

Diversify your lower-body workout routine by incorporating various exercises targeting different muscle groups. Include squats, lunges, leg presses, calf raises, and hamstring curls.

Periodically introduce new exercises to keep your routine engaging and prevent adaptation plateaus.

Warm-Up and Cool Down

Prioritize a thorough warm-up before engaging in lower-body exercises. This should include dynamic stretches and light cardiovascular activities to elevate your heart rate and prepare your muscles for the upcoming workload.

Incorporate static stretches during your cool-down to enhance flexibility and assist in recovery.

Progressive Overload

Implement the principle of progressive overload to challenge your lower-body muscles continually. Gradually increase your exercises' intensity, duration, or resistance over time.

This gradual progression stimulates muscle growth, strength development, and overall improvement in fitness.

Mix Strength and Functional Training

Combine traditional strength-training exercises with functional movements that replicate daily activities. This integration enhances muscle strength, coordination, balance, and joint stability.

Functional exercises may include step-ups, squats with overhead presses, or lunges with twists.

Include Bodyweight and Resistance Training

Integrate a mix of bodyweight exercises and resistance training to target different aspects of lower-body fitness.

Bodyweight exercises, like bodyweight squats and lunges, serve as foundational movements, while resistance training with weights or resistance bands adds progressive resistance for continued challenges.

Focus on Form and Range of Motion

Prioritize proper form during lower-body exercises to reduce the risk of injury and maximize effectiveness.

Ensure a full range of motion in each exercise, allowing muscles to be fully activated throughout the movement. This attention to form enhances muscle engagement and overall benefits.

Recovery and Rest Days

Plan for sufficient recovery time between lower-body workout sessions to allow muscles to repair and grow.

To aid recovery and prevent overtraining, incorporate rest days or engage in light activities like walking or gentle stretching on these days.

Listen to Your Body

Pay close attention to your body's signals during and after lower-body exercises. If you experience pain, discomfort, or fatigue, modify the exercises accordingly.

It's crucial to distinguish between muscle soreness, which is normal, and pain, which could indicate an issue requiring attention.

Functional Integration

Tailor your lower-body exercises to align with your fitness goals and daily activities.

If your goal is improved walking or enhanced athletic performance, choose exercises directly contributing to these objectives. Consider movements that improve balance, stability, and agility.

Consider Professional Guidance

Consult a fitness professional or physical therapist if you're new to exercise or have specific health concerns.

They can assess your fitness level, tailor a lower-body workout plan to your individual needs, and provide guidance on proper form, progression, and exercise modifications.

Incorporating lower-body exercises into your routine demands a thoughtful and strategic approach. By considering these detailed aspects, you can create a comprehensive lower-body workout plan that promotes strength, mobility, and overall fitness.

Long-Term Benefits

Strength in Daily Movements

Lower-body exercises, such as squats, lunges, and leg presses, target key muscle groups, such as the quadriceps, hamstrings, and glutes.

Strengthening these muscles improves the ability to perform daily tasks like standing up from a chair, getting in and out of a car, and lifting groceries.

Enhanced Balance and Stability

Exercises focusing on balance, such as single-leg stands or stability lunges, strengthen the stabilizing muscles around the ankles, knees, and hips.

Improved balance reduces the risk of falls, which is a common concern for older adults, and it also contributes directly to long-term independence.

Joint Flexibility and Range of Motion

Lower-body exercises involve dynamic movements that enhance joint flexibility and overall range of motion.

Improved joint flexibility is crucial for bending to tie shoelaces, reaching for items on low shelves, and maintaining fluid mobility.

Fall Prevention and Injury Mitigation

Strong lower-body muscles and improved balance significantly reduce the risk of falls.

In the long term, preventing falls is essential for avoiding injuries, fractures, and hospitalizations, thus supporting sustained independence.

Preservation of Bone Density

Weight-bearing exercises, such as walking and resistance training for the lower body, stimulate bone remodeling and help maintain bone density.

Over the years, preserving bone density has become particularly important in preventing fractures and maintaining skeletal health.

Joint Health and Arthritis Management

Regular lower-body exercises contribute to joint health by promoting synovial fluid circulation and strengthening the muscles that support the joints.

This is beneficial for managing arthritis and maintaining mobility, which is critical for long-term independence.

Cardiovascular Health Support

Dynamic lower-body exercises elevate the heart rate and contribute to cardiovascular health.

A strong cardiovascular system is vital for maintaining stamina and endurance, allowing for sustained physical activity and independence.

Functional Independence in Activities of Daily Living (ADLs)

Strengthening lower-body muscles directly impacts the ability to perform ADLs such as walking, climbing stairs, and getting in and out of a bathtub or shower.

Functional independence in these activities fosters self-sufficiency and long-term autonomy.

Improved Gait and Walking Ability

Lower-body exercises positively affect gait patterns and walking ability.

Maintaining a steady and efficient gait is crucial for staying mobile, reducing the risk of mobility-related issues, and ensuring independence in movement.

Reduced Risk of Chronic Conditions

Engaging in lower-body exercises is associated with a lower risk of chronic conditions, such as heart disease and diabetes.

Managing these conditions contributes to overall health and helps maintain mobility over the long term.

Positive Impact on Mental Well-being

Regular lower-body exercises release endorphins, improving mood and reducing stress.

Positive mental well-being is linked to a more active lifestyle, supporting long-term engagement in physical activities and maintaining independence.

Autonomy in Activities Requiring Lower-Body Strength

Long-term autonomy is fostered by maintaining lower-body strength, allowing for continued participation in gardening, recreational walking, and community engagement.

The ability to independently engage in these activities contributes to a fulfilling and independent lifestyle.

Focusing on lower-body exercises provides a targeted approach to preserving strength, balance, and mobility. These exercises address specific muscle groups and movement patterns that are essential for daily living, contributing significantly to long-term independence and overall well-being. Regular attention to lower-body fitness investments sustains autonomy and an active lifestyle.

Aspects to Remember

Consultation with a Healthcare Professional

Before starting any exercise program, especially for seniors with pre-existing health conditions, it's crucial to consult with a healthcare professional to ensure safety and suitability.

Start Gradually

Begin with low-intensity exercises and gradually progress to more challenging ones in order to avoid overexertion and reduce the risk of injury.

Proper Warm-Up

Always perform a thorough warm-up, including light cardio and dynamic stretches, to prepare the muscles and joints for the exercises.

Maintain Proper Form

Focus on maintaining correct form during exercises to prevent strain on joints and muscles. Consider seeking guidance from a fitness professional.

Use Support if Needed

To prevent falls, seniors can use support, such as a sturdy chair or railing, especially during balance-focused exercises.

Listen to Your Body

Pay attention to any discomfort or pain. If an exercise causes pain, it should either be modified or avoided. Seniors should listen to their bodies and not push through pain.

Stay Hydrated

Proper hydration is essential. Seniors should drink water before, during, and after exercise, especially if they are on medications that may cause dehydration.

Avoid Overexertion

Seniors should avoid overexertion and know their limits. It's crucial to pace oneself and take breaks as needed in order to prevent fatigue.

Breathing Technique

Practice controlled breathing during exercises. Avoid holding your breath, as proper oxygen flow is crucial for energy and muscle function.

Regular Health Checkups

Regular health checkups are essential for monitoring overall health. Any change in health conditions should be communicated to healthcare professionals.

Modify as Needed

Seniors should not hesitate to modify exercises based on their fitness level or any physical limitation they may have.

Choose Appropriate Footwear

Wear supportive and comfortable footwear to provide stability and reduce the risk of slips or falls during exercises.

Balance Exercises with Recovery

Allow sufficient time for recovery between exercise sessions to prevent fatigue and minimize the risk of injury.

Adapt to Physical Changes

Seniors should adapt exercises to accommodate any physical change or limitation they may experience due to aging or health conditions.

Environmental Considerations

Ensure the exercise environment is safe and free of hazards. Remove obstacles or loose rugs that may pose a tripping risk.

Chapter 5: Core Stability and Balance

Staying active is super important for staying healthy both mentally and physically. Nowadays, there are tons of new ways to move your body that are changing how people think about exercise, even for older folks. One technique that is gaining traction is core stability, which is basically about combining breathing and movement to strengthen your body's center.

You might picture hardcore athletes like boxers or skiers focusing on core workouts, but surprise! Pros from all sports, even soccer and softball players, swear by it. And hey, strong core muscles aren't just for athletes; they're handy for everyday stuff like sitting up straight, walking steady, and even catching that train without tripping. As you age, your bones weaken, your muscles shrink, and your balance isn't as sharp. This combo can make simple tasks harder and increase the risk of falls.

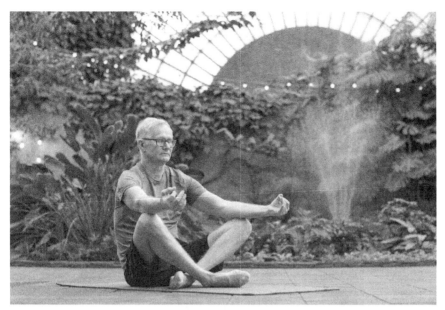
This combo can make simple tasks harder and increase the risk of falls.
https://www.pexels.com/photo/man-practicing-yoga-6787408/

To avoid that, it's crucial to keep your body strong and flexible with regular exercise, especially focusing on your core. This area, basically the middle part of your body, plays a key role in keeping you stable and preventing falls. Now, let's break down what core stability really means. It's about how well your diaphragm, abs, and pelvic floor work together to support your spine when you move.

Mastering core stability can help prevent injuries and pains, making it a smart move for anyone into sports or just staying active. Messing it up, though, can lead to back problems, especially if you're not careful with your movements. In simple terms, your core is your body's stabilizer, keeping your hips and chest steady and helping your muscles work efficiently.

So, why is having a strong core such a big deal? Well, it turns out that it's pretty crucial for our everyday lives, offering a bunch of benefits. First off, these core muscles are the body's support system for the spine, helping you move around safely and maintain good posture. They're the ones that handle any wobbles or imbalances that happen when you're on the move. One of the biggest perks? Core strength can help ease back pain, which is a common issue for many folks due to the heavy lifting your back muscles and bones endure. Having a strong core isn't just about looking good; it's about feeling good and moving better in your daily life.

Chair Jumping Jacks

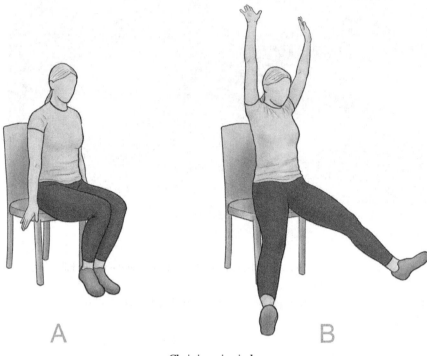

Chair jumping jacks.

Chair jumping jacks are a seated exercise that targets multiple muscle groups, including the core, shoulders, and legs. This exercise mimics the traditional jumping jack motion but is performed while seated on a chair, making it suitable for individuals with limited mobility or those who prefer a low-impact workout.

Instructions:

1. Sit up straight in a sturdy chair with your feet flat on the floor, hip-width apart.
2. Keep your arms relaxed at your sides.
3. As you inhale, simultaneously lift your arms out to the sides and above your head while spreading your legs out to the sides.
4. Exhale as you bring your arms back down to your sides and close your legs together.
5. Perform 10 full repetitions, focusing on maintaining a smooth and coordinated motion.

6. Keep your core engaged throughout the exercise to support your spine and stabilize your body.

Modified Version:

To make chair jumping jacks easier, perform the exercise at a slower pace and with smaller movements. You can also start by lifting only your arms or legs at a time instead of both simultaneously.

Ab Twists

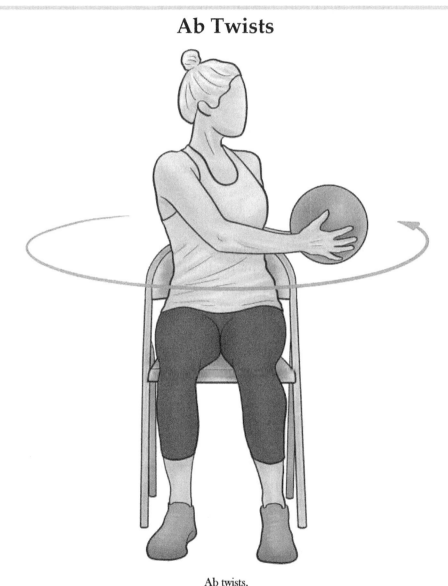

Ab twists.

Abs twists are an effective exercise for targeting the obliques, which are the muscles on the sides of your abdomen. This exercise also engages the core muscles and improves stability and balance. By using a medicine ball or similar object, you add resistance to the movement, making it more challenging and effective for strengthening the abdominal muscles.

Instructions:

1. Sit on the outer edge of a chair with your feet flat on the floor and your knees bent at a 90-degree angle.

2. With both hands, hold a medicine ball in front of your chest while bending your elbows.

3. To keep your spine stable and your posture correct, contract your core muscles.

4. Bring the medicine ball towards your right hip by slowly rotating your torso to the right.

5. After going back into the center, twist to the left to move the ball closer to your left hip.

6. Continue alternating sides for a total of 10 repetitions (5 twists to each side).

7. Focus on controlled movements and exhale as you twist to engage your abdominal muscles more effectively.

Modified Version:

If using a medicine ball feels too challenging, you can perform abs twists without any weight or with a lighter object, such as a water bottle. You can also reduce the range of motion by twisting your torso only slightly from side to side, gradually increasing the range as you build strength.

Forward Bend in a Chair

The forward bend in a chair is a gentle stretching exercise that primarily targets the hamstrings, lower back, and shoulders. It helps improve flexibility in the spine and hamstrings while also promoting relaxation and reducing tension in the upper body.

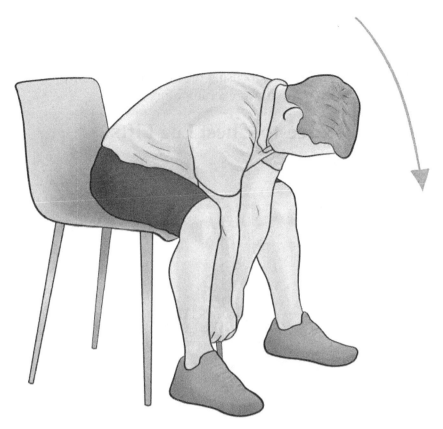

Forward Bend in a Chair.

Instructions:

1. Sit tall in a chair with your feet flat on the floor, hip-width apart.

2. Inhale deeply and extend your spine.

3. Lean forward from your hips and extend your hands as far down as is comfortable, or toward the floor, as you release the breath.

4. Let your head swing freely, and let your neck loosen.

5. Feel a light stretch in the lower back and back of your legs as you hold the pose for a few breaths.

6. Inhale as you slowly return to an upright position, bringing your arms back up alongside your body.

7. Exhale and repeat the forward bend, syncing your movements with your breath.

8. Continue for 10 repetitions or as long as it feels good, gradually increasing the depth of the stretch over time.

Modified Version:

If reaching toward the floor is too challenging, you can place your hands on your thighs or knees instead. You can also perform the exercise with a lesser range of motion, focusing on maintaining good posture and feeling a gentle stretch without overexerting yourself.

Knee-to-Chest Leg Lifts

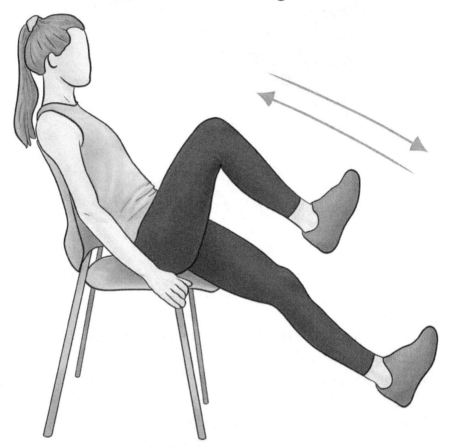

Knee-to-chest leg lifts.

Knee-to-chest leg lifts target the lower abdominal muscles, hip flexors, and quadriceps. This exercise promotes better posture and balance and helps to increase hip joint flexibility, stability, and core strength.

Instructions:

1. With your feet flat on the ground and your knees bent 90 degrees, take a seat on the edge of a chair.

2. To stabilize your spine, tighten your core muscles and hold onto the chair's sides for support.

3. Extend both legs in front of you with your toes pointing up toward the ceiling.

4. While keeping your back straight, slowly lift one knee toward your chest as high as comfortable, maintaining balance and control.

5. Hold the position for a few seconds, feeling the contraction in your lower abdomen.

6. Slowly lower your leg back down to the starting position.

7. Repeat the movement with the opposite leg.

8. Continue alternating legs for a total of 8 to 12 repetitions, focusing on controlled movements and breathing.

Modified Version:

If lifting both knees simultaneously is too challenging, you can start by lifting one knee at a time while keeping the other foot firmly planted on the floor for added stability.

Extended Leg Raises

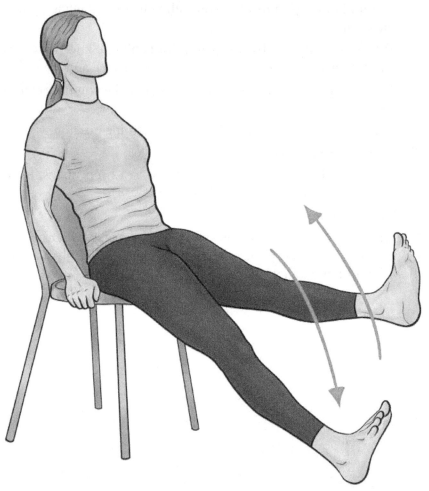

Extended leg raises.

These focus on the quadriceps, hip flexors, and lower abdominal muscles. This exercise promotes better posture and balance and helps to increase hip joint flexibility, stability, and core strength.

Instructions:

1. With your feet flat on the floor and your knees bent 90 degrees, take a seat on a chair's edge.

2. To keep your posture upright and your chest open, contract your core muscles.

3. For balance, grip the chair's sides.

4. With your toes pointed skyward, extend your legs diagonally in front of you.

5. Lift one leg slowly as high as you can while keeping your body stable and your core tight.

6. Hold the lifted position for a few seconds, feeling the contraction in your lower abdomen and hip flexors.

7. Return the raised leg to its starting position gradually.

8. Repeat the movement with the opposite leg.

9. Each leg lift counts as one repetition.

10. Aim to complete 12 repetitions in total, focusing on controlled movements and breathing.

Modified Version:

If lifting both legs simultaneously is too challenging, you can start by lifting one leg at a time while keeping the other foot firmly planted on the floor for added stability.

Chair Backbend

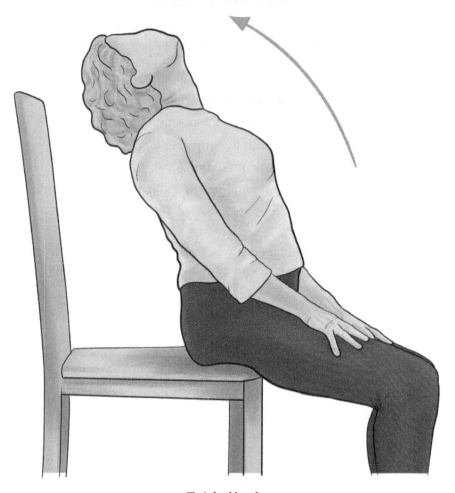

Chair backbend.

The chair backbend is a gentle stretching exercise that primarily targets the chest, shoulders, and upper back. It helps improve flexibility in the spine and shoulders while also promoting relaxation and reducing tension in the upper body.

Instructions:

1. With your feet flat on the ground and your knees bent at 90 degrees, take a comfortable seat on a chair's edge.
2. Keep your spine straight, and your shoulders relaxed.
3. Place your hands on your hips for support.

4. Slowly lean back with your upper body, arching your spine gently.

5. Allow your chest to open up and your stomach to protrude slightly forward.

6. Hold the stretch for 10 to 20 seconds, focusing on deep breaths and relaxing into the stretch.

7. Slowly return to an upright position, bringing your spine back to neutral.

8. Repeat the stretch 5 times, gradually increasing the duration of each stretch as it feels comfortable.

Modified Version:

If leaning back is too challenging, you can place a cushion or pillow behind your back for support. You can also perform the stretch while sitting further back in the chair with your back supported by the chair's backrest.

Bending to the Side

Bending to the side is a seated stretching exercise that primarily targets the obliques and lateral muscles of the torso. This exercise helps improve flexibility in the side body and promotes better posture and spinal alignment.

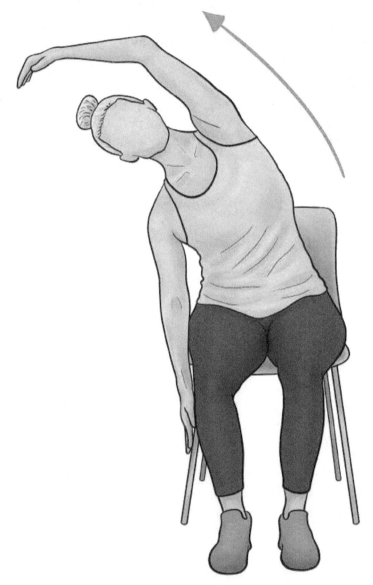

Bending to the side.

Instructions:

1. With your feet flat on the ground and your knees bent at 90 degrees, take a comfortable seat on a chair's edge.

2. Keep your spine tall, and your shoulders relaxed.

3. Raise your right arm overhead, bending it at the elbow, and allow your left arm to hang by your side.

4. Inhale deeply, lengthening your spine.

5. As you exhale, slowly bend to the left side from your waist, sliding your left hand down your leg toward the floor.

6. Keep your chest open and your right elbow gently pulling back to feel a stretch along the right side of your body.

7. Feel the right side gently lengthen as you hold the stretch for a few breaths.

8. Breathe out as you raise yourself back up and put your arms in the initial position.

9. Repeat the stretch on the opposite side, raising your left arm overhead and bending to the right side.

10. Perform 12 repetitions in total, alternating sides with each repetition.

Modified Version:

If reaching toward the floor is too challenging, you can place your hand on your hip or thigh instead of reaching toward the floor. You can also perform the stretch with a lesser range of motion, focusing on the lateral movement of your torso without straining.

Forward Roll-Ups in a Seated Position

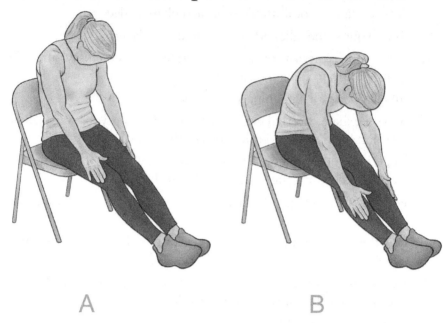

Forward roll-ups in a seated position.

Forward roll-ups in a seated position are a core-strengthening exercise that primarily targets the abdominal muscles. This exercise helps improve core stability, posture, and spinal alignment.

Instructions:

1. Sit tall in a chair with your legs stretched out in front of you, your heels on the ground, and your feet flexed.

2. Place your hands in front of you on the chair for support and to maintain good posture.

3. Inhale deeply, lengthening your spine and engaging your core muscles.

4. Exhale slowly, bringing your chin toward your chest and rolling your torso forward over your thighs.

5. Reach your hands toward your toes as far as comfortable, feeling a stretch along your spine and hamstrings.

6. Inhale as you slowly roll back up to an upright position, stacking your spine vertebra by vertebra.

7. Repeat the movement with controlled and deliberate breaths, focusing on engaging your abdominal muscles throughout the movement.

8. Perform 8 repetitions in total, maintaining a smooth and controlled motion.

Modified Version:

If rolling all the way forward is too challenging, you can start by rolling halfway down and then back up to an upright position. You can also perform the exercise with your hands resting lightly on your thighs for added support.

Seated Torso Twists

Seated torso twists are a seated exercise that targets the oblique muscles, which are the muscles on the sides of your abdomen. This exercise strengthens the core muscles and enhances spinal flexibility and mobility.

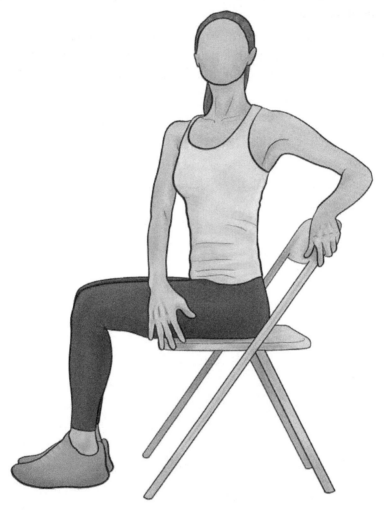

Seated torso twists.

Instructions:

1. Take a comfortable seat on the edge of a chair, keeping your knees bent at a 90-degree angle and your feet flat on the ground.
2. Grip the sides of the chair for support.

3. Use your core muscles to keep your spine stable and your posture correct.

4. Slowly twist your torso to the right, bringing your left hand toward the outside of your right thigh or knee.

5. Feel the muscles on the left side of your torso gently lengthen as you hold the twisted position for a short while.

6. Return to the center and then twist your torso to the left, bringing your right hand toward the outside of your left thigh or knee.

7. Feel the muscles on the right side of your torso gently lengthen as you hold the twisted position for a short while.

8. Repeat the movement, alternating between sides for a total of 10 repetitions on each side.

9. Focus on controlled movements and avoid twisting too far to prevent strain on your spine.

Modified Version:

If twisting your torso fully is too challenging, you can perform the exercise with a lesser range of motion by twisting only to a comfortable position without forcing the stretch. You can also perform the movement at a slower pace, focusing on engaging your core muscles throughout the exercise for stability and support.

Seated Side Reaches

Seated side reaches are a core and balance exercise that targets the obliques and improves lateral stability. This exercise can aid with core strengthening and improving sitting balance.

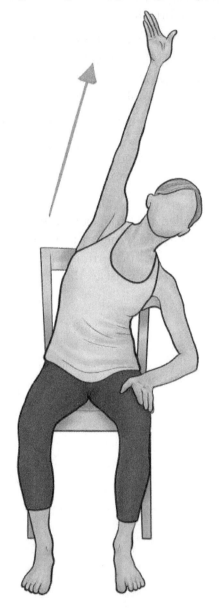

Seated side reaches.

Instructions:

1. Sit comfortably on the edge of a chair with your feet flat on the floor and your knees bent 90 degrees.

2. Throughout the workout, contract your core muscles to keep your spine stable and your posture correct.

3. Extend your arms out to the sides at shoulder height, with your palms facing down.

4. Inhale deeply and lengthen your spine.

5. Exhale slowly as you lean to one side, reaching toward the floor with your hand.

6. Keep your opposite hand lifted and reaching overhead to elongate the side of your body.

7. Feel a light stretch along the side of your torso as you hold the stretched position for a few seconds.

8. Inhale as you return to an upright position.

9. Repeat the movement on the opposite side, leaning toward the other side and reaching toward the floor.

10. Continue alternating between sides for a total of 10 to 12 repetitions on each side.

11. Focus on controlled movements and maintaining proper posture throughout the exercise.

12. Keep your core engaged, and avoid leaning forward or backward in the chair.

Modified Version:

If reaching toward the floor is too challenging, you can perform the exercise with smaller movements by reaching toward your knee or thigh instead. Simply lean to one side and reach toward your knee while keeping the opposite hand lifted overhead, alternating between sides.

Seated Torso Twists with Resistance Band

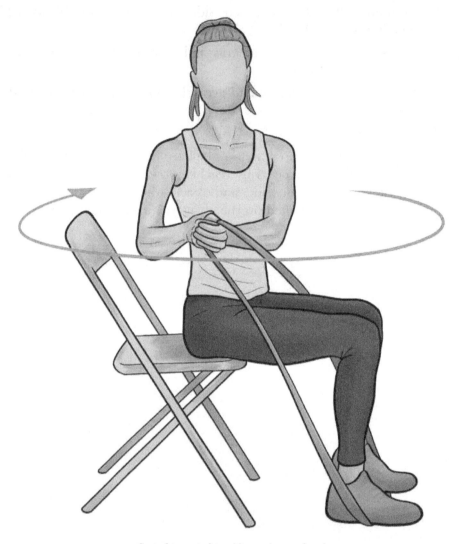

Seated torso twists with a resistance band.

Seated torso twists with a resistance band are excellent for targeting the obliques, improving spinal mobility, and enhancing core stability. This exercise helps to strengthen the muscles responsible for twisting movements and promotes better balance while seated.

Instructions:

1. Sit comfortably in a chair with your feet flat on the floor and your back straight.
2. Secure one end of a resistance band under your foot and hold the other end with both hands, positioning it at chest level.
3. Engage your core muscles to stabilize your spine and maintain good posture throughout the exercise.
4. Exhale as you twist your torso to one side, pulling the resistance band across your body.
5. Keep your arms extended and rotate your shoulders, feeling the contraction in your oblique muscles.
6. Inhale as you return to the starting position, resisting the pull of the band and controlling the movement.
7. Repeat the twist on the opposite side, pulling the resistance band across your body in the opposite direction.
8. Continue alternating between sides for a total of 10 to 12 repetitions on each side.
9. Focus on controlled movements and maintaining proper posture throughout the exercise.
10. Keep your core engaged, and avoid leaning forward or backward in the chair.

Modified Version:

If using a resistance band is too challenging, you can perform the exercise without any equipment by simply twisting your torso from side to side while seated.

Seated Leg Extensions with Stability Ball

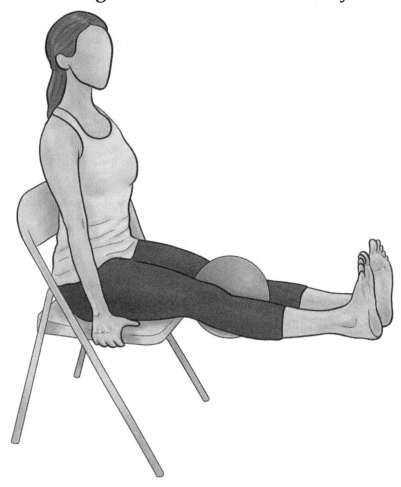

Seated leg extensions with a stability ball.

Seated leg extensions with a stability ball are effective for targeting the core muscles, particularly the lower abdominals, while also improving balance and stability. This exercise helps to strengthen the core and promote better posture while seated.

Instructions:

1. Sit comfortably in a chair with your feet flat on the floor and your back straight.

2. Place a stability ball between your knees and engage your core muscles to stabilize your spine.

3. Hold onto the sides of the chair for support, if needed.

4. Exhale as you extend your legs out in front of you, squeezing the stability ball between your knees.

5. Hold the extended position for a few seconds, focusing on maintaining your balance and engaging your core muscles.

6. Inhale as you bend your knees and return to the starting position, bringing the stability ball back toward your body.

7. Repeat the leg extensions for 10 to 12 repetitions, focusing on controlled movements and maintaining proper form.

8. Keep your core engaged throughout the exercise to support your lower back and promote better posture.

9. Avoid arching your back or leaning backward in the chair.

Modified Version:

If using a stability ball is too challenging, you can perform the exercise without any equipment by simply extending one leg at a time while seated. Focus on engaging your core muscles and performing controlled movements to maximize the benefits of the exercise.

These exercises will not only strengthen your core muscles but also improve your stability, posture, and mobility while seated. Whether using resistance bands, stability balls, or simple bodyweight movements, consistent practice of these exercises can lead to better balance, reduced risk of falls, and improved quality of life, especially for older adults with limited mobility or those who spend extended periods sitting.

Chapter 6: Mind and Body Connection: Mindfulness and Breathing Techniques

The purpose of mindfulness is to bring focus to the task at hand, making it an essential component of any exercise regimen. This chapter outlines the benefits of mindfulness and breathing techniques for mental clarity, stress reduction, and overall well-being. It also comes with a few exercises (along with step-by-step instructions and tips) you can use to practice mindfulness.

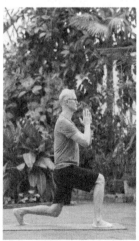

The purpose of mindfulness is to bring focus to the task at hand.
https://www.pexels.com/photo/man-practicing-yoga-6787357/

For added benefits, the chapter offers suggestions for integrating mindfulness and breathing techniques into your chair exercise practice and daily life. Lastly, you'll read about the holistic benefits of combining physical exercises with mental training in more detail.

The Benefits of Mindfulness and Breathing Techniques

Mindfulness and breathing techniques have long been known for their holistic benefits.

They Help Regulate the Nervous System

Consisting of a bundle of nerves, the autonomic nervous system is responsible for specific reactions to the stimuli in the environment, known as "rest and digest." Mindfulness exercises (especially mindful breathing) foster the activation of this state, allowing the body and mind to reach a state of calmness. Moreover, deep breathing helps activate the logical part of the brain, enabling you to execute good decision-making skills and rational thinking even in stressful times.

They Bring Pain Relief

Living with chronic pain can make it hard to focus on everyday tasks, let alone workouts. Mindfulness exercises can take your mind off of pain, decrease your discomfort, and make physical activity easier. It does this by helping deactivate activity in the thalamus — the pain-processing center of your brain.

They Help Chase Away the Worries

The amygdala — the tiny, almond like structure at the back of your brain, is responsible for emotional control responses. When the amygdala becomes active, it triggers the fight or flight response, putting your body in a state of distress. Slow, deep, and controlled breathing can reduce activity in the amygdala, signaling that there is no stress to cope with.

Mindful breathing also reduces the release of dopamine and other stress-related biochemicals in your body, which fosters better stress response. These hormones are activated when you feel anxious or fearful and the physical signs of stress appear. Activating the rest-and-digest state counteracts the effects of the stress-induced amygdala activation.

They Help You Sleep Better

Ever had trouble falling asleep, having your mind filled with worries about the future or memories of the past? Or, perhaps, you find yourself waking up several times through the night. Then, you feel fatigued throughout the day and lack the energy to perform daily activities. Sleep deprivation also affects your ability to focus during exercise. This is because stress, pain, and other factors detrimental to health reduce melatonin production. Melatonin is essential for a good night's sleep, and mindful breathing can help stimulate its production.

They Improve Physical Health

Beyond the benefits for your mental and emotional health, mindfulness and breathing techniques also have a positive impact on your physical health. For one, the different aspects of your health are connected, so by improving one, you can improve them all. For example, if you feel anxious or overwhelmed, your heart rate increases, and your breathing becomes shallow. You're taking more oxygen into your body, and the nutrients aren't getting into your organs because your circulation becomes compromised. These are all-natural stress responses in the body that can be managed through mindful breathing and other mindfulness exercises. If not, the long-term effects of these stress-induced symptoms can be detrimental to your physical and mental well-being. They can even affect your physical performance during exercise. Taking deeper, controlled breaths can reduce your heart rate, return your circulation to its normal rhythm, and supply enough oxygen to your body.

Improving your circulation can also boost your cognitive functions, which will help you focus on your workouts and everyday tasks better. Moreover, it will lower your risk of cardiovascular diseases, type 2 diabetes, cortisol spikes, and more.

Similar to aerobic exercise, regular, mindful, deep breathing can improve your lung capacity, enabling you to breathe properly even through the most demanding moments.

Mindfulness exercises can even improve digestion by providing more oxygen to your gastrointestinal tract. Your body will be able to absorb more nutrients to keep you healthy, and your immune system will be stronger to keep away infections.

They can Improve your Mental Health

Mindful breathing and other mindfulness techniques are excellent ways to get in touch with the sensations in your body. While doing this, you no longer focus on whatever you are worried about or have negative thoughts about yourself or something else. It helps the unwanted negativity fade away, helping you improve your mental health. Either as part of other mental health interventions or as standalone exercises, mindfulness and breathing techniques can help manage the symptoms of anxiety and depression, anger, emotional turmoil, and psychological symptoms of emotional or physical trauma. It can also help combat the psychosomatic effects of chronic pain.

Mindfulness and Breathing Techniques for Seniors

Belly Breathing

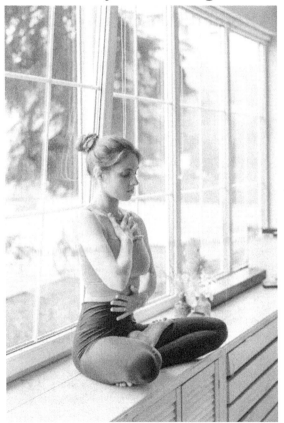

Belly breathing.

https://www.pexels.com/photo/a-woman-in-beige-tank-top-sitting-near-the-glass-windows-while-meditating-4534856/

Belly breathing can help you strengthen the muscles in the diaphragm, enabling you to breathe deeper and become stronger during exercise, stress, or simple everyday activities.

Instructions:

1. Sit tall in a comfortable position. Close your eyes or soften your gaze — whatever you prefer.
2. Place your right hand on your chest and your left one on your belly.
3. Take a slow, deep breath through your nose and feel how your belly expands.
4. As you release the breath, feel how your belly falls.
5. Do this breathing technique for 5 to 10 minutes once a day.

Alternate Nostril Breathing

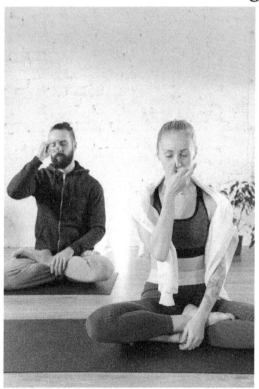

Alternate nostril breathing.
https://www.pexels.com/photo/a-man-and-a-woman-meditating-practicing-breathing-control-6648542/

This ancient breathing form facilitates simultaneous relaxation in the mind and body.

Instructions:

1. Sit or lie down on a yoga mat, keeping your back straight. Close your eyes or soften your gaze — whatever you prefer.

2. Cut off the airflow at your left nostril with your left thumb.

3. Inhale through your right nostril. When your belly has expanded, close your right nostril with your right ring finger.

4. Hold your breath for a few seconds.

5. Open up your left nostril and exhale through it.

6. Then, inhale through your free nostril again, close it, and free the other one to exhale through it.

7. Keep alternating between the nostrils for 5 to 10 minutes.

4-7-8 Breathing

If stress hinders you from relaxing before exercise or during the day, this breathing technique will bring you the calmness you need.

Instructions:

1. Sit or lie down on a yoga mat. Close your eyes or soften your gaze — whatever you prefer.

2. Take a deep breath through your nose while counting to four.

3. Hold your breath while counting to seven.

4. Slowly exhale while counting to eight.

5. Do 4 to 8 repetitions twice a day — once when you feel stressed throughout the day and once before going to bed.

Pursed Lip Breathing

This simple breathing technique can boost your lung function, making it easier to breathe during physical activities.

Instructions:

1. Sit or lie down with your back straight and your shoulders relaxed.

2. With your mouth closed tightly, take a deep breath through your nose while counting to two.

3. Imagine you are about to blow out a candle and purse your lips.

4. Slowly release your breath through your puckered lips while counting to four.

5. Do the exercise for 5 to 10 minutes a day.

Box Breathing

Box breathing is another fantastic tool for enhancing your focus.

Instructions:

1. Find a comfortable position. You can stand, sit, or lie down.

2. Close your eyes and imagine you're standing on top of a square box.

3. Take a deep breath while counting to four and imagining you're moving toward the side of the square box.

4. Hold your breath while counting to four and moving toward the bottom of the square box in your mind.

5. As you exhale and count to four again, you can see yourself moving toward the other side of the square box.

6. Hold your breath while counting to four and imagine yourself reaching the top of the square box again.

7. Try going around the square for 5 to 10 minutes every day.

Quick Body Scan

A quick body-scan meditation will help you become aware of your body's sensations, explore their origins, and devise your workout routines accordingly.

Instructions:

1. Find a quiet space where you can relax. It's best if you sit or lie down, but you can remain standing if you wish.

2. Close your eyes and deepen your breathing.

3. As you breathe deeply, notice how each part of your body feels. Start at your toes and examine every part of yourself systematically until you reach the crown of your head.

4. Have you noticed tension anywhere? If so, how can you relieve it?

Connecting with Nature

Connecting with the natural world around you is one of the easiest ways to enhance your mental well-being.

Instructions:
1. Find a calm patch of nature and take a few moments to stand or sit in it.
2. Take a few breaths and take note of your surroundings.
3. What can you pick up in each of your senses? Take time to appreciate all this.

Five Senses

This mindfulness exercise is a great way to ground yourself in the present moment and focus your attention on the world around you. You can do it anywhere, anytime. And it's a great way to bring your attention back to the present when feeling stressed or overwhelmed.

Instructions:
1. Start by closing your eyes and taking a few deep breaths.
2. Then, begin to notice what you're experiencing through your senses. Can you notice five things you can see, four things you can feel, three things you can hear, two things you can smell, and one thing you can taste?
3. Work on noting all this for complete relaxation in your mind and body.

Gratitude Exercise

Practicing gratitude is another superb exercise that fosters mindfulness. You can use it to cultivate this skill, focus on the positive aspects of your life, and spend less time with worrisome thoughts that may affect your physical and mental health.

Instructions:
1. Take a few minutes to think about or write down things you're grateful for. These can include your health, family, and friends, as well as your favorite possessions.
2. Focusing on what you're grateful for can help you appreciate the good in your life and make it easier to let go of negative thoughts

and emotions. It can be easy to get bogged down in the negative aspects of life - especially when things are tough.

Creative Mindfulness

Ever found yourself doodling something while on the phone with someone? Creating art is an underrated mindfulness technique you can easily incorporate into your life. It doesn't have to be anything complex or fancy. Even a 10-minute mindful drawing exercise will go a long way to clear your mind. Suppose you don't feel like getting creative with drawing or other forms of art. In that case, you can always use a coloring book instead and just let your imagination loose on the shades you want to use.

Instructions:

1. Sit tall with your shoulders relaxed.
2. Take a deep breath in for five seconds, and then breathe out slowly for five seconds. Repeat this up to ten times.
3. As you pick up your tool, note your grip. Is it too tight or too loose? Feel free to try different ways of holding it until you find the one that helps you relax.
4. Then, switch your focus on what you want to create. You can draw inspiration from music by playing your favorite songs, describing the emotions you're feeling at the current moment, depicting a person of your choice or a silhouette, or looking outdoors from a window or while on your latest walk.

Integrating Mindfulness Techniques into Your Chair Exercise Practice and Daily Life

Approaching health goals with a more mindful perspective could offer a better solution for long-term success because it helps you to be fully present when you need to make healthy choices. This is why integrating mindfulness into your chair exercise regime will enable you to get the most out of it. Try checking in with yourself after your chair exercise each day to see how you feel. Then, try doing this on the days you don't work out.

However, the art of mindfulness can also be useful in daily life. Mindfulness is all about being present, and you can be present at any time — when washing the dishes, walking your dog, or taking a bath.

One of the best ways to incorporate mindfulness and breathing techniques into your exercise is to learn to stay present during workouts. Your goal is to go through the movements with the utmost intent to stay in good form and alignment. Sometimes, your mind suddenly starts to wander. This is normal, and everyone experiences it from time to time. The key is to understand how to bring it back to the present. Being fully present is particularly crucial for improving balance and posture, building muscle, and fostering recovery from injury or an illness. So, next time your mind travels off mid-exercise, focus on engaging your muscles and feeling their contraction. With practice, your focus will improve, along with the quality and effectiveness of your workout. You can do the same when you find yourself losing focus on a task or chore you're doing.

Breathing has a surprisingly vast impact on exercise. Yet, many people simply forget to breathe because they focus too much on getting the movement right. Focusing on breathing fosters proper muscle engagement and coordination, ultimately maximizing the movement's effectiveness. When engaging and contracting your muscles, always take a deep breath. As you release it, you should expand and release the muscles.

Breathing techniques can also come in handy when you feel stressed or anxious. For example, the Breath of Peace is a powerful exercise that focuses on controlling breathing. Deep, conscious breathing not only oxygenates the brain but also slows the heart rate, imbuing a sense of calmness. Whenever you feel stressed, inhale deeply through your nose, pause, and exhale slowly, releasing your stress, along with the air from your lungs. Continue until you feel your mind return to its balanced state. You can also incorporate this exercise into your daily routine. For instance, you can do it before going to bed at night. You'll fall asleep faster and have better sleep quality through the night.

Mind to Your Fitness Habits

To establish new habits that foster better exercise results, you must be aware of the decisions you're making throughout the day. This is an automatic process, and unless you bring awareness to it, you'll likely experience a detour. For example, do you give priority to doing the chair exercises every day? Or do you tend to put off your workouts, intending to pick up the routine later? If the second one applies, be mindful of your intention to fight off the urge to postpone your workouts. For example, when you wake up in the morning, write down on a piece of paper, "I will exercise today, no matter how I feel about it." If you need to, keep looking at the paper until it's time to get moving. This is just to help you focus on your intention. Later, thoughts of working out will pop up automatically throughout the day.

Fully Experience the Present

Sometimes, mindfulness is simply taking the time to appreciate each moment. For example, at any point of the day, you can stop and look around, absorbing the shapes and colors of everyday objects. Or, you can take your time while cooking and consuming a meal, savoring the scents and flavors and identifying the individual aromas mixed in the flavor combination. You can also explore the sensation while sitting and watching TV, standing in line at the grocery store, or walking. Active listening is another fantastic tip — it helps you tune into the sounds around you as well as the conversations you are having with others.

Mindful Walking

Walking is probably one of the simplest acts of mindfulness that has ever existed, yet it has a plethora of benefits. Try paying attention to the rhythm of your walking and the sensation coursing through your body when you walk. Let your surroundings become your focal point, and you'll see why. Since it combines physical activity with mindfulness, walking is particularly beneficial for seniors.

The Holistic Benefits of Combining Physical Exercises with Mental Training

Combining physical exercises with mental training can benefit you in many wonderful ways, including the ones listed below.

Improved Focus

Ever catch yourself taking long breaks between sets, getting distracted with thoughts of everyday tasks? Mindful breathing throughout the exercise can help you remain focused on maintaining proper form and alignment, avoid sudden movements that could lead to injuries, and eliminate distractions. Being fully present during workouts will allow you to pay undivided attention to what you're doing.

Advanced Body Awareness

Practicing mindfulness is an excellent way to get in touch with your body. By getting to know your body, you become more cognizant of the sensations coursing through it during exercise.

Gentle movements for seniors are designed to be done slowly, which fosters a greater focus on breathing — not just because honing in on your breath means you can shut out worries. It makes it easier to notice your form and correct it if necessary, and feel if a movement causes tension in any area and adjust it accordingly. This will go a long way in preventing exercise-related injuries, which are more common in the elderly.

Better Mental Health

If you aren't used to physical exercise, it takes unremitting motivation to stick with any workout routine. One of the reasons why many people fail to stay motivated to work out is because they become overly stressed about performance and results. Mindfulness is an excellent stress reliever, with the ability to chase away any worry that would interfere with your fitness plans. By practicing breathing and other mindfulness techniques, you can learn to be patient and solely focused on getting a little better every time, which will give you a confidence boost and motivate you to keep moving.

Greater Enjoyment

If you have mobility issues, then physical activity will be the last thing you think will bring you joy. Mindfulness can help you change this belief. By allowing you to be fully present and in the moment, it will show you all the things you can appreciate about your physical activity — the sound of your breath supplying your body with oxygen, the movements your muscles are capable of, and the beauty of your surroundings. Moreover, mindfulness and breathing exercises can teach you how to become more aware of your progress, which will make the workouts even more enjoyable.

Chapter 7: Flexibility and Mobility: Stretching and Movement

Maintaining good physical health is key, and flexibility plays a crucial role. As you go through life, various factors like aging, sitting for too long, or poor posture can chip away at your flexibility. Imagine sitting at your desk for hours on end, feeling your muscles tighten up like an old rubber band, or trying to tie your shoes and realizing you can barely reach your toes anymore – that's the reality for many people!

This is where chair yoga comes in. It gives your body a much-needed tune-up and helps you stretch out those tight muscles and grease the joints. Yoga isn't just about physical flexibility; it's a stress-buster, too. Think about those moments when life throws one too many curveballs your way, and you feel like you're carrying the weight of the world on your shoulders.

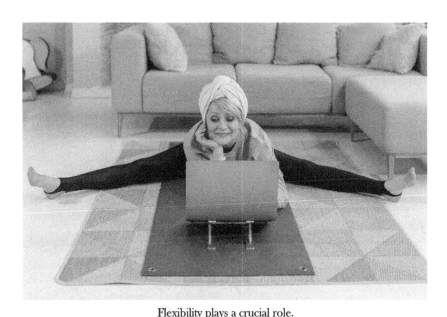

Flexibility plays a crucial role.
https://www.pexels.com/photo/person-people-woman-relaxation-7530023/

This chapter is tailored to address the specific needs of older adults seeking to regain flexibility and mobility. These accessible poses are designed to accommodate varying levels of flexibility and mobility, providing a gentle yet effective means of improving overall physical well-being. Whether you're recovering from a sedentary day at the office or looking to counteract the effects of aging, these chair yoga poses will help you reclaim freedom of movement in your life.

Latissimus Stretch

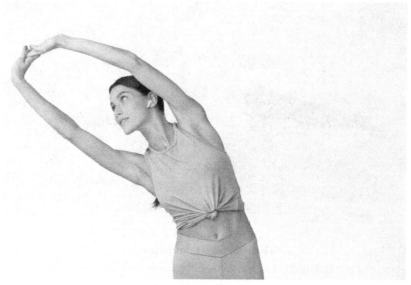

Latissimus stretch.

This exercise targets the latissimus dorsi muscle, which is crucial for upper-body flexibility and posture.

Instructions:

1. Stand by a chair, holding its back or its seat with your left hand for support.

2. Extend your right arm overhead, reaching toward the ceiling with your palm facing away. Aim for full extension without straining.

3. Imagine pulling your right shoulder higher for an added stretch.

4. Keep your back straight and engage your core.

5. Hold for 20 seconds, feeling the stretch in your right side, ribs, and under your armpit.

6. Release and lower your arm.

7. Repeat on the other side, using your right hand on the chair and stretching your left arm overhead.

Modified Version:

To make this stretch easier, perform it while seated in the chair. Sit comfortably with a straight back, then raise one arm overhead while holding onto the chair's armrest for support. Feel the stretch in your side and ribs without overexerting yourself.

Stretching the Wrist Flexor

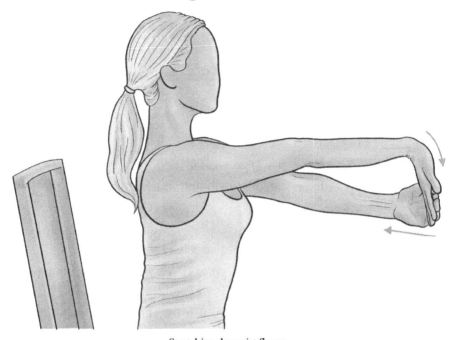

Stretching the wrist flexor.

This exercise stretches the muscles of the forearm and wrist, promoting flexibility and relieving tension.

Instructions:

1. Sit comfortably in your chair with a straight back.
2. Extend your right arm in front of you, palm facing down.
3. Use your left hand to gently pull back the fingers of your right hand toward your body.
4. Feel a stretch along the forearm and wrist.
5. Hold for 15 to 30 seconds, then switch to the other arm.

Ankle Movements

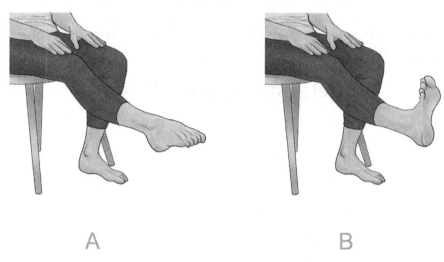

A   B

Ankle movements.

Ankle movements enhance ankle flexibility and circulation in the lower limbs.

Instructions:

1. Sit with your back against the chair's backrest.
2. Lift one foot slightly off the floor and flex your toes, bringing them up toward your shin.
3. Point your foot forward, curl your toes, and then straighten them out.
4. Repeat this process on your other foot.
5. Perform 10 repetitions on each ankle, emphasizing controlled movements to enhance flexibility.

Seated Neck Turns

This exercise promotes neck mobility and relieves tension in the cervical spine.

Instructions:

1. Sit comfortably with your hips back and your back supported by the chair.
2. Maintain a straight spine and upright posture for core stability.
3. Plant both feet firmly on the ground.
4. Slowly turn your head right or left for a gentle stretch.
5. Hold for 30 seconds, then switch directions.
6. Repeat 3 to 5 times in each direction.

Modified Version:

For a gentler stretch, sit comfortably in the chair with an upright posture. Gently turn your head to one side, holding for 20 to 30 seconds, then switch to the other side. Repeat as desired for a soothing neck stretch.

Mountain Pose in a Chair

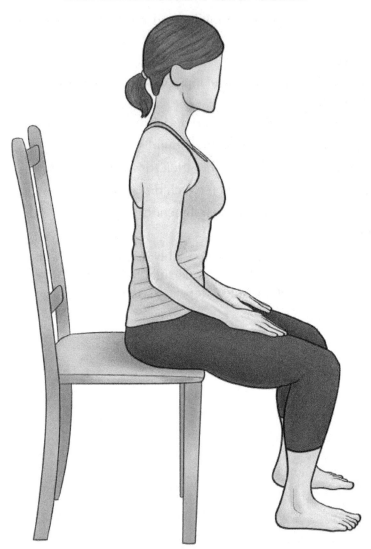

Mountain pose on a chair.

This seated variation of the mountain pose promotes alignment and core stability.

Instructions:

1. Sit in the chair's center, keeping your upper body relaxed and upright. Sit on your sit bones for stability, adjusting your buttocks slightly outward.

2. Place your hands on your lap, maintain an upright torso, tuck in your tailbone, and draw your belly button toward your spine. Keep your shoulders and neck relaxed, facing forward.

3. For comfort and alignment, roll your shoulders back, broaden your chest, and lower your shoulder blades.

4. Position your feet hip-width apart, aligning your heels with your knees.

Modified Version:

If you feel uncomfortable, use support like a bolster or a blanket, ensuring it's not too thick. This maintains even weight distribution and lets you feel your sit bones on the support, enhancing stability during the pose.

Variation #1

Instructions:

1. Interlace your fingers and gently press against your jawline, tilting your gaze upward.

2. Relax your fingers, move them to the back of your head, and apply gentle pressure to bring your chin closer to your chest.

Variation #2

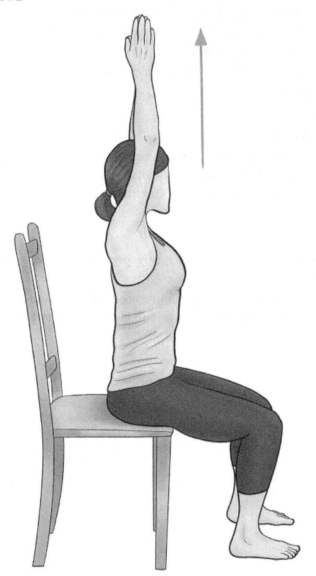

Mountain pose on a chair.

Instructions:

1. Return to the mountain pose, then extend your right arm overhead, reaching toward the ceiling.

2. Incline your head to the right, clasping your left ear with your outstretched hand.

3. Straighten your left arm alongside your left thigh until you feel a stretch in the left side of your neck.

4. Repeat on the opposite side, reaching your left hand to grasp your right ear and straightening your right arm.

Variation #3

Instructions:

- Begin in the mountain pose with your head bowed.

- Slowly rotate your head in a complete circle, circling to the left twice. Repeat the circular motion in the opposite direction.

Forward Bend with Two Chairs

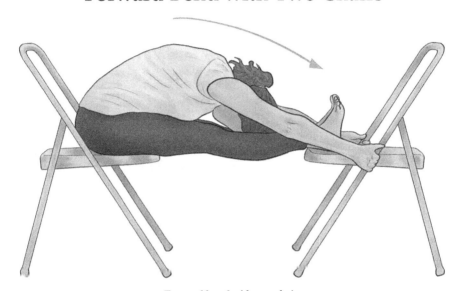

Forward bend with two chairs.

Instructions:

1. Set up two chairs of equal height facing each other, with a leg's length apart.

2. Sit on one chair, extending your legs onto the other, ensuring your knees are fully straightened and your feet stay flat on the seat.

3. Flex your feet, keeping your toes pointed upward.

4. Inhale, reaching both arms overhead with your fingers extended.

5. Exhale slowly, folding your torso forward and resting your lower abdomen on your upper thigh, maintaining good spinal alignment.

Depending on flexibility:

- Place your hands on the thighs, knees, ankles, or soles of your feet without compromising spine straightness.

- Alternatively, grab the sides of the spare chair for extra support if needed.

Modified Version:

For a gentler stretch, sit on the edge of one chair with your feet flat on the floor. Extend your arms forward, then slowly hinge at the hips and lean forward, allowing your torso to rest on your thighs. Hold for a comfortable duration, feeling the stretch in the lower back and hamstrings.

Feet Stretching

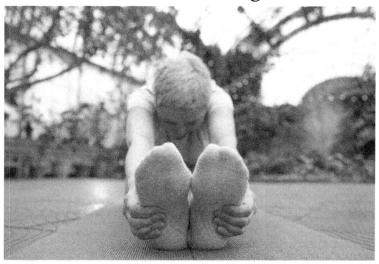

Feet stretching.

https://www.pexels.com/photo/woman-stretching-her-body-forward-6787441/

Instructions:

1. From the mountain pose, roll your ankles inward, grazing your soles on their outer edges. Hold for a few breaths, then return to start.

2. Shift your weight forward with your heels rising and your toes bearing the load. Sway them playfully side to side.

3. Press your heels down, reach your toes skyward, and tuck under your metatarsals for a gentle stretch.

4. If comfortable, lift your heels to enhance the pull.

Hugging Knees

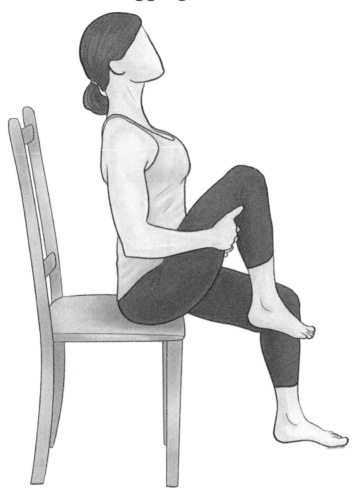

Hugging knees.

Instructions:

1. Sit upright in your chair with your arms by your sides.
2. Draw one knee up toward your chest, holding the shin or thigh for balance.
3. Keep the other leg planted on the floor.
4. Hold for five deep breaths, maintaining a straight spine.
5. Slowly lower the knee back to the mountain pose and repeat with the other leg.

Fingers Interlocking and Back Bending

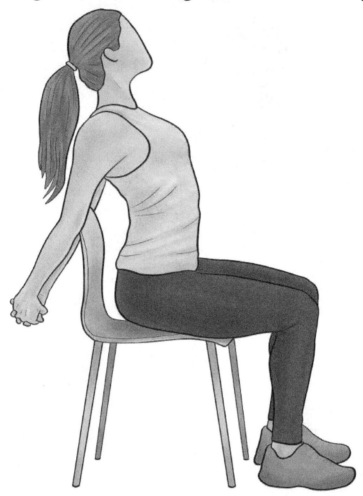

Fingers Interlocking and Back Bending.

Instructions:

1. Begin in the mountain pose with a straight back.

2. Interlace your fingers behind your lower back, ensuring a secure lock before straightening your elbows.

3. Look upward, lifting your chest and feeling a stretch in your arms and shoulder blades.

4. For an added challenge, slightly bend forward and raise your interlaced arms overhead.

Eagle Pose in a Chair

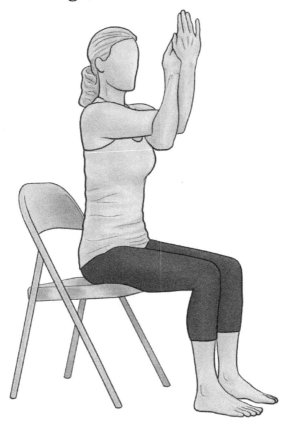

Eagle Pose in a Chair.

Instructions:

1. Sit comfortably upright in your chair with a straight back and relaxed shoulders.

2. Extend your arms in front at chest height, elbows bent at 90 degrees, and fingers pointing up.

3. Stack your right elbow atop the left, allowing your hands to naturally cross.

4. Interlace your fingers, even if your right hand only reaches the tips of the left fingers.

5. Inhale deeply, lifting both elbows and bringing your upper arms perpendicular to your chest.

6. Exhale slowly, relaxing back to a neutral position.

Seated Forward Bend

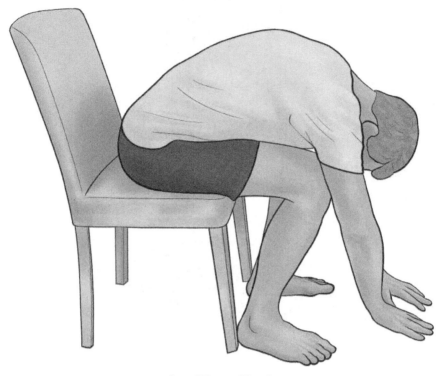

Seated Forward Bend.

Instructions:

1. Sit tall in your chair with your feet slightly wider than hip-width apart.

2. Inhale deeply, lengthening your spine, and reach your arms up toward the ceiling.

3. Exhale, bending forward from your lower waist and folding your torso between your thighs.

4. Softly rest your shoulders on your knees or keep your arms extended forward for good spinal alignment.

5. Hug the shins with your hands, or hold your arms outstretched.

6. Hold for at least five deep breaths, enjoying the back and hamstring stretch.

Downward Facing Dog (Modified)

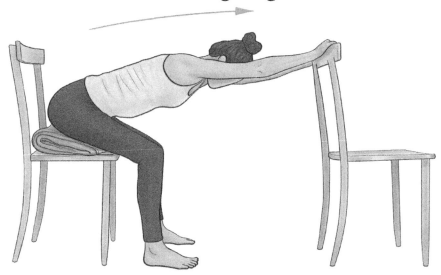

Downward Facing Dog.

Instructions:

1. Grab two chairs. Place the second chair with the backrest facing you, about an arm's length away. Adjust the distance for your leg length.

2. Start in the mountain pose with your feet hip-width apart and your arms by your sides.

3. Inhale and raise your arms overhead, lengthening your spine.

4. Exhale slowly and bend your torso forward, reaching your hands toward the backrest.

5. Keep your back straight, engage the core, and lengthen your spine.

6. Hold this position, enjoying the gentle chest and shoulder stretch. Breathe deeply and focus on relaxation.

Chair Pose (Modified)

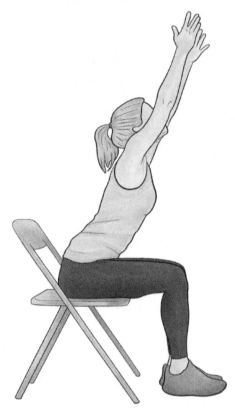

Chair pose.

Instructions:

1. Return to the mountain pose with your feet hip-width apart and your arms by your sides. Inhale deeply, raising your arms overhead and reaching toward the ceiling to lengthen your spine.

2. Exhale slowly, and begin to fold your torso forward, aiming for a 45-degree angle. Focus on engaging your core and maintaining a long, straight spine.

3. Hold for 5 deep breaths, focusing on breathing and enjoying the gentle back stretch.

4. Inhale, and slowly rise back to the mountain pose with your arms at your sides.

5. Repeat this fold several times for a complete set.

Sun Salutation in a Chair

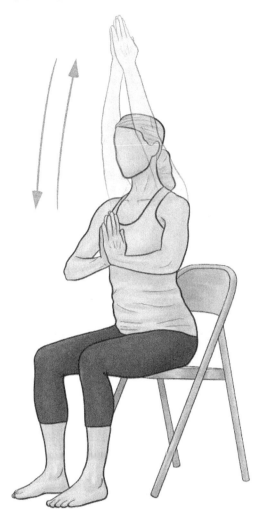

Sun salutations.

Instructions:

1. Sit comfortably with your spine straight.
2. Inhale, reaching your arms overhead with your palms facing each other.
3. Exhale, bringing your hands to the heart center.
4. Inhale again, extending your arms back overhead.
5. Repeat this flow, coordinating each movement with your breath.

Bear Hug

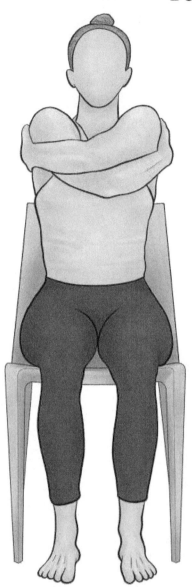

Bear hug.

Instructions:

1. Sit comfortably in your chair, maintain good posture, and inhale deeply.

2. As you exhale, open your arms wide, sweeping them around in a bear-hug motion, embracing yourself.

3. Cross your arms in front of your chest, allowing your shoulder blades to gently separate.

4. Inhale as you expand your chest, and exhale as you release the hug.

5. Repeat this sequence, connecting your breath with the comforting bear-hug motion.

Goddess Pose in a Chair

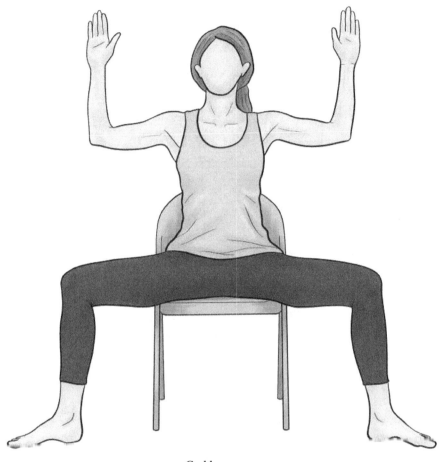

Goddess pose.

Instructions:

1. Sit comfortably in the chair's center with your feet wide on the floor, experiencing a gentle stretch in the inner thighs and hips.

2. Extend your arms to the sides, keeping your elbows straight and parallel to the floor, with your palms facing forward.

3. Bend your elbows upward, forming 90-degree angles between your upper and lower arms, envisioning your arms in a welcoming embrace.

17. Modified Camel Pose

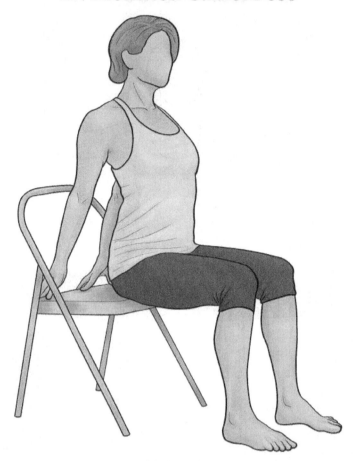

Modified camel pose.

Instructions:

1. Sit up with your feet hip-width apart, facing the chair. Move the seat forward slightly if comfortable.

2. Place your fingertips behind your lower back, near the spine base.

3. Roll your shoulders back and down, unfolding like a flower.

4. Curve back forward, puffing your chest up comfortably.

5. Keep the neck muscles relaxed, and gaze upward or forward without tensing your shoulders.

6. Maintain a round position for five deep breaths, feeling a gentle stretch in the lower back and chest openness.

7. Slowly unwind the spine to a neutral, straight-back position.
8. Pause, breathe, and feel the release before optionally repeating on the opposite side.

Seated Fish Pose

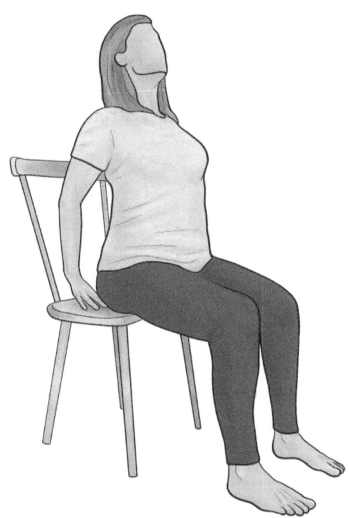

Seated fish pose.

Instructions:

1. Begin in the mountain pose.
2. Move toward the front edge of the chair, leaving space behind for your hands.

3. Reach back, placing your fingertips near the base of your spine.
4. Inhale deeply.
5. Exhale, pressing your fingertips into the chair as you lift your chest and imagine your spine lengthening.

Choose your depth:

- For a shallower bend, gently tuck your chin; for a deeper backbend, gaze softly upward.
- Hold for several seconds, taking five slow breaths into your rib cage.

Seated Figure 4 Stretch

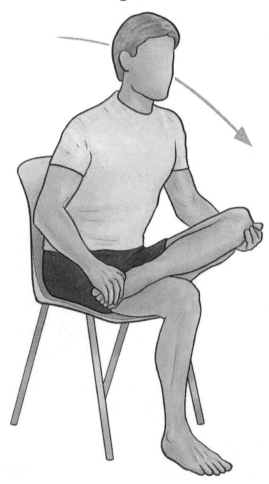

Seated figure 4 stretch.

Instructions:

1. Maintain an upright posture in your chair.
2. Cross your right ankle over your left knee, creating a "figure 4" shape with your legs.
3. Keep your back straight and gently lean forward, feeling a stretch in the outer hip and glutes.
4. Hold the position for 20 to 30 seconds before switching to the other leg.

Modified Boat Pose

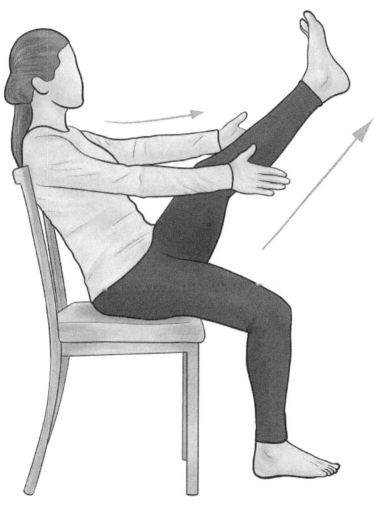

Modified boat pose.

Instructions:

1. Sit on the edge of the chair, allowing room to lean back at a 45-degree angle while keeping your chest upright. Ensure stability.

2. Hold your right knee behind you, pulling it close to your chest while maintaining an upright position. Hold a straight leg raise and pointed toes.

3. Release the knee, extend your arms forward, and engage your core while gently squeezing your hamstring to maintain the pose.

4. For an added challenge, lift your other leg for a bird-like balance. Alternatively, switch legs and repeat the sequence.

Half Lord of the Fish Pose

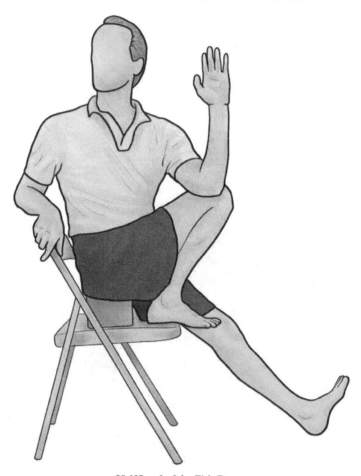

Half Lord of the Fish Pose.

Instructions:

1. Stand in the mountain pose.
2. Extend your left leg straight forward, flexing your foot and engaging your toes.
3. Bend your right knee and bring your ankle toward your left groin.
4. Inhale deeply and raise your arms to lengthen your spine.
5. Exhale slowly and twist your torso to the left.
6. Reach your right hand to the outer sole of your left foot.
7. Hold for five breaths.
8. Release and repeat these steps on the opposite side.

Seated Noose Pose

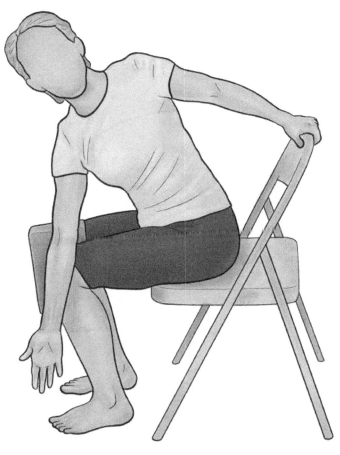

Seated Noose Pose.

Instructions:

1. Sit tall in a chair with your feet flat on the floor, hip-width apart (the mountain pose).
2. Take a big breath and lift both arms above your head.
3. Exhale, lower your right arm, reaching across to the left side of your left thigh.
4. Choose your left arm option:
5. Beginner: Keep your left arm stretched toward the ceiling.
6. Advanced: Reach your left arm behind and grab your right waist.
7. Gently press your right elbow into the outside of your left knee to deepen the twist.
8. Breathe and hold for a few breaths.
9. Open your chest by rolling your right shoulder back and down for a deeper stretch. Keep your gaze upward.

Seated Tortoise Pose

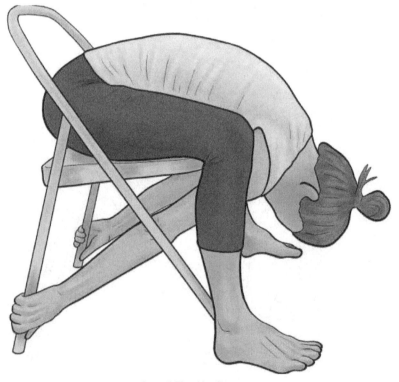

Seated Tortoise Pose.

Instructions:

1. Sit tall in a chair with your feet flat on the floor, hip-width apart. This is the mountain pose.
2. Slide your bottom slightly forward on the chair.
3. Open your legs wider than hip-width apart.
4. Inhale deeply and lengthen your spine.
5. Exhale slowly and fold your torso forward, keeping your back straight.
6. Reach your hands down toward the floor between your legs.
7. Gently drag your hands back through the gap between your legs.
8. Choose one option for your hands:
9. Grab the chair legs for support.
10. Place your hands flat on the floor just outside your feet.

Chair Race

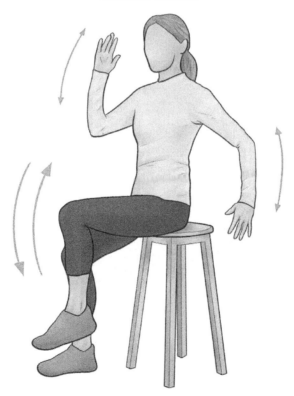

Chair race.

Instructions:

1. Sit tall in your chair with your arms relaxed at your sides.
2. Bring your right knee up toward your chest as you turn your left shoulder down to meet the right knee.
3. Simultaneously, bend your left arm at the elbow.
4. Return to the starting position and bring the left knee up to meet the right shoulder, pumping your right arm.
5. Repeat these alternating motions, creating a seated "running" motion.
6. Execute 10 to 20 repetitions for each leg, focusing on the rhythmic and controlled movements.

Ankle Stretching

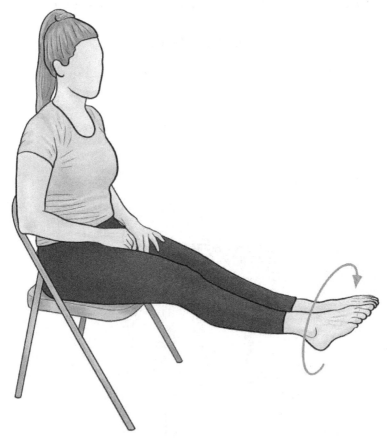

Ankle Stretching.

Instructions:

1. Sit tall in a chair with your feet flat on the floor. Lift both legs slightly off the ground, just a few inches.

2. Make small, smooth circles with your ankles, moving in both directions. Imagine you're drawing tiny circles with your toes.

3. Squeeze your toes as you make the circles. This helps stimulate the muscles and nerves in your feet.

4. Continue for 10 to 15 circles in each direction.

5. Repeat with the opposite leg.

Seated Bicycle Pedaling

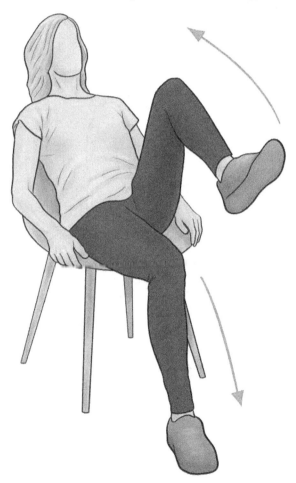

Seated Bicycle Pedaling.

Instructions:

1. Sit in the chair with your back against the backrest and your feet flat on the floor.
2. Hold onto the chair's edge for stability.
3. Lift your right leg as high as possible with your knee bent, mimicking a pedaling motion.
4. Return your right foot to the floor, repeating the process with your left leg.
5. Perform 10 repetitions for each leg, focusing on the fluidity of the circular motion and engaging your core for stability.

Elbow to the Alternate Knee Switch

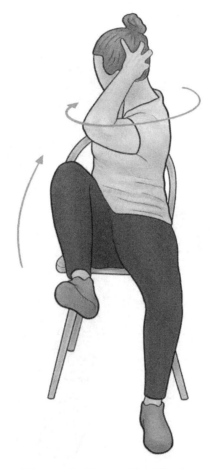

Elbow to the Alternate Knee Switch.

Instructions:

1. Begin seated with a straight back and your feet flat on the floor.
2. Place your right hand behind your head, creating a sharp angle with your arm.
3. Raise your left knee and rotate your right elbow, bringing it toward your left knee.
4. Repeat this movement 10 times. Switch sides, using your left elbow and right knee, and perform an additional 10 repetitions.
5. Maintain a controlled pace throughout.

Seated Child Pose

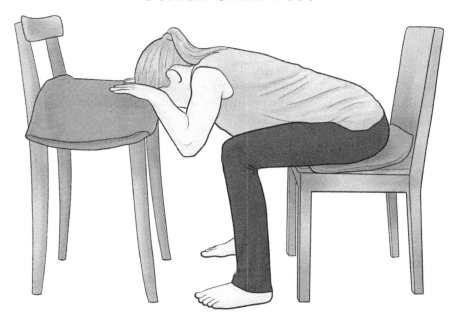

Seated child pose.

Instructions:

1. Use two chairs — one for sitting comfortably, the other for hand support in your forward bend.
2. Make the second chair cozy with a blanket or a pillow.
3. Sit tall with your feet flat and your back straight.
4. Inhale, raise your arms overhead, and stretch toward the ceiling.
5. Exhale, gently fold forward, and rest your head on the pillow or chair.

6. Find a comfortable hand position on the seat or draped over the back.

7. Relax in this position, enjoying the stretch and taking a mini vacation for your body and mind.

8. Keep your elbows slightly bent and your spine lengthened — no slouching!

9. Focus on deep inhales and slow exhales, imagining the tension washing away like gentle waves. If reaching the floor is hard, sit on the chair's edge. Add more pillows for head support.

10. For a neck stretch, tilt your head to one side, holding for a few breaths. Repeat on the other side, releasing tension like sails unfurling.

Make sure to incorporate these poses into your daily routine so that you can effectively address common issues like stiffness, tension, and poor posture that may arise from prolonged sitting or a sedentary lifestyle. Whether you're at home, in the office, or traveling, these accessible and adaptable practices allow you to prioritize self-care and maintain a healthy body and mind.

Chapter 8: Restorative Practices: Gentle Movements for Recovery

Whether you're having a laid-back day, recovering from injury or surgery, or looking to rebuild your strength and independence gently, there are a variety of easy-to-perform chair exercises that suit your individual needs.

The aim of these restorative practices is not exclusive to physical abilities – they also work on stabilizing the mental state and improving overall well-being. Besides the basic strength exercises, there are other, more holistic-based ones, better known as chair yoga.

Many people picture yoga as a complicated, physically taxing exercise that requires a lot of flexibility. This idea is far from the truth. Chair yoga is a practice that does not rely too much on the practitioner's physical ability but helps to rebuild and stabilize the body through a slow, stable, and measured pace.

Other variations of exercises can be applied during recovery besides chair yoga. As you venture through this chapter, you'll learn how to restore balance and strengthen your body with simple, safe, and easy-to-perform exercises.

Chair Yoga

This type of yoga has become a fan favorite among people of all ages, and especially seniors, due to its accessibility and economical nature. You don't need any equipment to perform these exercises. All you need is a chair, which is a very common household item that's easy to come by.

There are many notable benefits to chair yoga. As you progress in these exercises, you'll notice an increase in overall flexibility and better balance.

The practice also helps with pain management, levels out your blood pressure, improves blood circulation, and doesn't put too much strain on the joints as most other exercises do. In addition to these benefits, there are mental benefits that include stress reduction and lowering the risk of depression and anxiety.

The beautiful thing about chair yoga is that you won't be restricted to following the regiment of one form of yoga. Instead, you'll find that the practice takes all the known forms of yoga and tailors them in a more accessible, chair-friendly way.

Getting Started

First, find a sturdy, straight-back chair to sit in. Before diving into the poses, begin with a simple meditation to clear out your mind and calm your breath. Sit still with your back straightened comfortably while engaging your core.

Take a deep breath, expand your chest, and then exhale, bringing down your shoulders and relaxing them. Repeat the breath, inhaling and exhaling the air with an equal count for a few minutes.

Overhead Stretch Pose

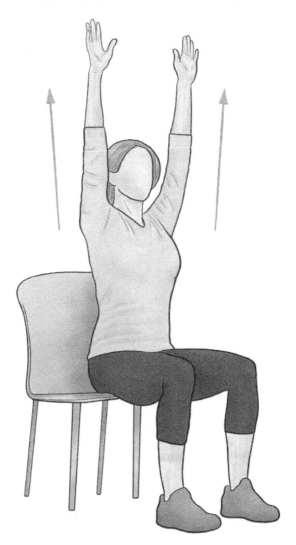

Overhead Stretch Pose.

1. This pose strengthens the obliques, latissimus dorsi, and deltoid muscles (sides, back, and shoulders).

2. To begin, take a seat with your back straight, face forward, and your arms by your sides.

3. As you slowly raise your arms toward the ceiling, take a deep breath in your chest.

4. Take a moment to hold your extended arms in place, then slowly release your breath as you lower them.

5. Continue in the same position, being careful to maintain a long, straight spine and to activate your core.

6. After a while of doing the exercise, you'll notice an improvement in your posture, breathing, and overall strength in your abdominal region.

Reverse Arm Hold Pose

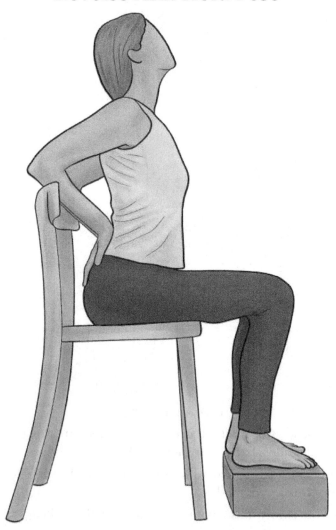

Reverse Arm Hold Pose.

1. This pose focuses on strengthening the arms and deltoids and stretching the spine.
2. Start by sitting upright in a straight-backed chair while keeping a small distance between your back and the back of the chair.
3. Place your arms at a wide, low angle on either side of your body, and take a slow, deep breath.
4. Breathe out slowly and gently. Then, begin to reach with your hands behind your back and slightly bend your elbows.
5. Maintain the same posture while gradually arching your back until your shoulders start to feel stretched.
6. Breathe deeply several times while holding this position, and then slowly raise your arms back to the starting position.
7. As you continue this practice, you will find that any muscle tension in your spine is released, with a noticeable improvement in your breath, posture, and stress levels.

Seated Forward Bend Pose

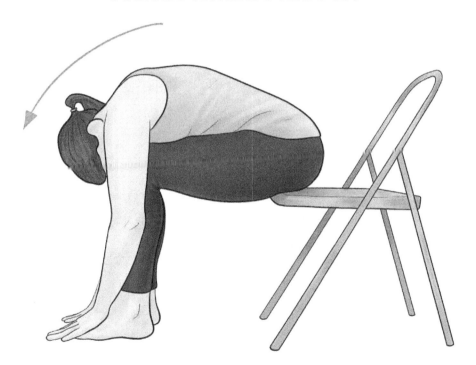

Seated Forward Bend Pose.

1. This position works on stretching the spine, torso, hips, and arms.
2. Start in a seated position with a straight back, knees held together, and feet planted firmly on the ground.
3. Inhale slowly and deeply through your nose. As you exhale the air, slowly start bending forward, focusing on the stretching sensation in your back.
4. Continue to lean forward as far as you can go without feeling any pain or discomfort in order to avoid injuries.
5. Hold in the furthest position you can get while taking several deep breaths, and then return slowly to the upright position you started with.
6. This position works on improving the performance of the digestive system, reducing the feeling of fatigue, and curing and preventing any lower-back pain while strengthening your posture.

Chair Warrior Pose

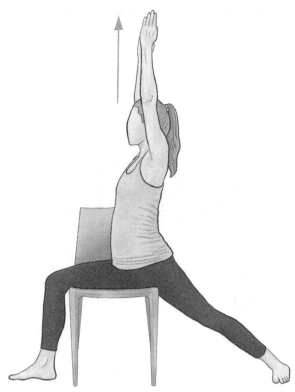

Chair Warrior Pose.

1. This exercise works on stretching several muscle groups, including the triceps, spine, trapezius muscle, abdominal muscles, deltoids, and Latissimus Dorsi.

2. Start this pose by sitting straight and facing forward while keeping your arms downward by your sides at a low and wide angle. In another variation of the exercise, start by lifting up your leg across the chair while keeping your torso stationary and facing forward. Do not attempt this technique unless you are confident in your flexibility or are being monitored by a professional for impromptu assistance.

3. Lift your arms high in the air and take a deep breath in.

4. Stay in your current form while performing deep, calming inhales and exhales. After a few moments, slowly return your arms to their original position.

5. While performing the other variation of this technique, remember to repeat the exercise with the other leg across the chair.

6. This pose promotes better posture and eases stress while calming your mind.

Chair Spinal Twist Pose

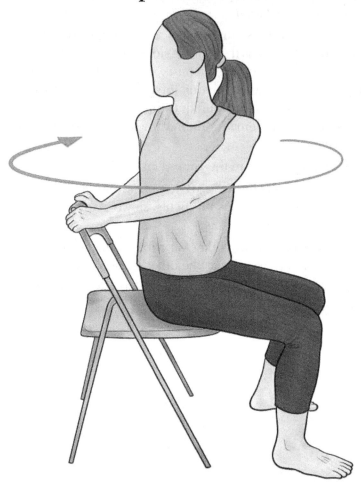

Chair Spinal Twist Pose.

This yoga pose works on stretching the spinal muscles and the pelvic muscles.

1. In this exercise, start with a sideways seated position in a sturdy chair. Place your legs on the right side of the chair, and make sure to keep your right arm rested next to the back.

2. Make sure your arm and body are not touching the back of the chair. Maintain a straight back and a proper posture.

3. Hold on tight to the chair's back with both of your hands, take a deep cleansing breath, and start gently and slowly turning your

body around to face the back of the chair. Make sure to let out your breath in a slow exhale.

4. While you're in a twist, make sure you've reached the farthest point possible without hurting yourself or feeling uncomfortable. Stay still, breathe in and out deeply, and then gently twist back and face forward again.

5. Make sure you're exercising both sides of your body equally. Turn your legs to the left side of the chair, keeping your left arm next to but not touching the back of the chair, and repeat the maneuver again.

6. This pose revitalizes organs, such as the kidneys and the digestive system, and improves overall flexibility.

Seated Mountain Pose

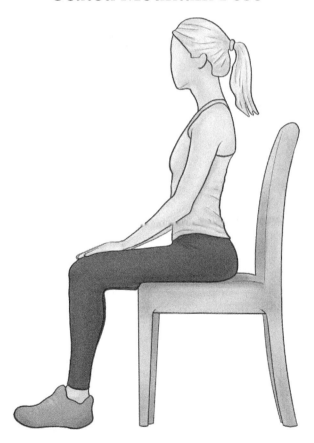

Seated Mountain Pose.

1. This position stretches the muscles in the arms, wrists, shoulders, and spine.
2. Starting with a straight back and an engaged core, go forward on the front part of the chair to begin the position.
3. Hold a 90-degree bend in your knees, keeping them level just above your ankles and allowing a small gap between them.
4. Inhale deeply and slowly, then begin to roll your shoulders downward as you exhale.
5. Hold your arms by your sides as you contract your abdominal muscles.
6. Keep the pose while inhaling and exhaling several times before returning to the original position.
7. This pose relieves pain in the muscles and relaxes strain in your body.

Cat-Cow Stretch Pose

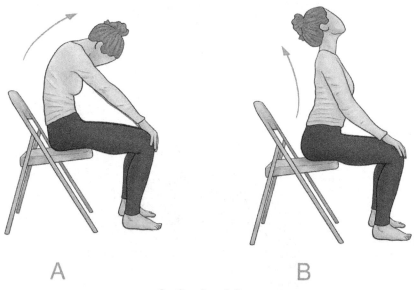

A   B

Cat-Cow Stretch Pose.

1. This position works on stretching the shoulders, abdomen, hips, and spine.
2. Keeping your hands on your knees and your back and spine straight, begin by sitting on the edge of your chair and using your core.

3. Inhale deeply, then begin the "cow stretch," which involves slowly and carefully arching your back as far as it will comfortably allow you to. For three to five deep breaths, hold this position.

4. After slowly bringing your back to its initial upright posture, begin the cat stretch by inverting forward.

5. Sustain the forward bend of your spine while positioning your shoulders above your hips.

6. Keep the position for a few deep breaths and then slowly return back to the upright position.

7. This exercise alleviates stress, engages and reinforces the organs in your abdomen, and increases flexibility in your spine.

Eagle Arms Pose

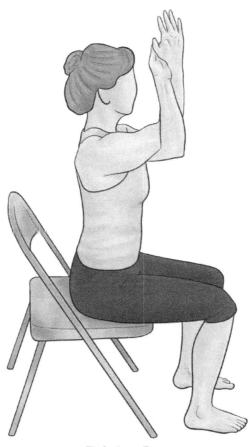

Eagle Arms Pose.

1. This pose stretches out the rotor cuff muscles, the deltoids, and the muscles in the arms.

2. When sitting, maintain an upright posture with your arms extended straight in front of you.

3. Begin by crossing your left arm across your right, and then pull your forearms closer together by bending your elbows.

4. After entwining your fingers, slowly elevate your elbows while slightly arching your back.

5. After holding the stance for a few slow, deep breaths, go back to the starting position.

6. Switch arms, placing your right arm over your left arm and repeating the exercise again.

7. This pose works on improving arm circulation, focus, and digestive activity.

Chair Pigeon Pose

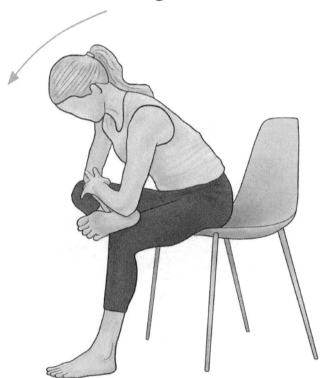

Chair Pigeon Pose.

1. This exercise works on stretching the hamstrings, pelvic muscles, hips, peroneus longus, and peroneus brevis (also simply known as the ankles).

2. Sit facing forward in your chair, with your back and spine straight and long, maintaining space between your back and the back of the chair.

3. Start raising your left ankle to rest upon either your right knee or thigh.

4. If you can't raise your ankle, you can lift it up with your hand.

5. Take a deep breath in and start flexing your left foot a little bit.

6. Bend forward a little bit and maintain your posture as you begin to softly exhale.

7. Breathe deeply for a few moments while you're still bent, and then slowly raise yourself back up to your starting posture.

8. Repeat the exercise by switching your legs and raising your right ankle to rest on your left thigh or knee.

9. This exercise improves overall posture and alignment, lessens lower back pain, and increases hip flexibility.

Neck Stretch Pose

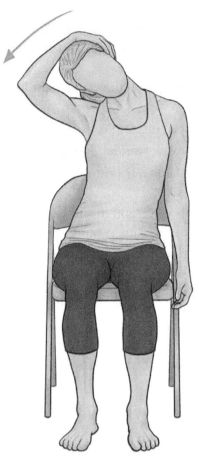

Neck Stretch Pose.

1. This pose targets the scalenus medius muscle, the trapezius, the levator scapulae, and the sternocleidomastoid muscle (basically all things neck-related and the upper center of the back).

2. You start by sitting up straight in your chair and leaving some distance between your back and the back of the chair.

3. Start to slowly extend your neck upward. You'll feel the sensation of the crown of your head moving toward the sky.

4. Reach up gently with your left hand to grasp onto your left temple while holding onto the base of your chair with your other hand.

5. Inhale deeply, and as you exhale, start to slowly move your left ear down toward your left shoulder. Try to fight the temptation to bend your back or raise your right shoulder up.

6. Hold your position while inhaling and exhaling several times.

7. Return to your original position and then repeat the movements on the other side of your body.

8. This exercise reduces any pain in the neck and also reduces stress, promoting a relaxed sensation throughout your body.

Triangle Pose

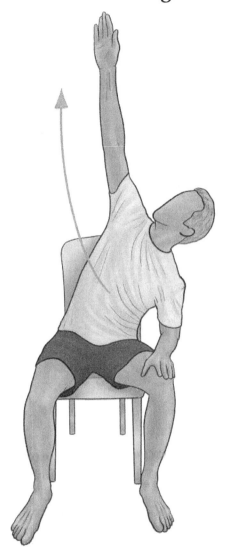

Triangle Pose chair.

1. This pose stretches several muscle groups, including the core, hamstrings, arms and shoulders, chest, and psoas, among others.

2. First, start by sitting upright on the edge of the chair. Face forward with your back straight.

3. Place your left hand on your left thigh with your fingers facing inward. Then, start to slowly and gently raise your right arm up toward the ceiling.

4. Lean gently forward with your torso, and start twisting your body toward your right shoulder, keeping your right arm and head facing the wall.

5. After taking a few deep breaths to hold the pose, carefully bring yourself back up to your starting upright position.

6. If you're unable to continue to hold your arm up, you can return it to your right hip while maintaining the right twist of your torso.

7. Repeat the exercise on the other side of your body.

Seated Overhead and Forward Stretch Pose

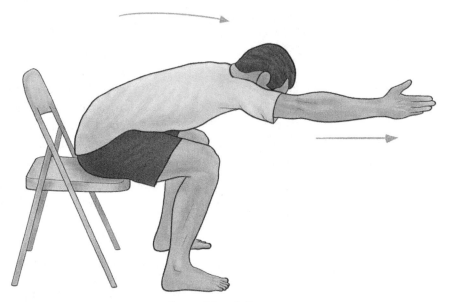

Forward Stretch Pose.

1. This exercise is completed in 2 parts, and it focuses on stretching the hamstrings, back muscles, and glutes.

2. Start by scooting forward and sitting on the edge of your chair while keeping your back and spine straight.

3. Inhale deeply, arch your back slowly and exhale as you begin to raise your right arm over your head.

4. Take another breath in, and while exhaling, start to bend forward as far as you can go with your right arm still stretched in front of your body.

5. Make sure your arm is right along your ear while maintaining the stretch.

6. Hold the pose while planting your feet firmly on the ground for a couple of deep breaths.

7. Return to the original position by keeping your arm stretched by your ear and straightening your back. Arch your spine once you're upright, and then bring your arm down slowly.

8. Repeat the exercise again for the other side of your body.

Other Strengthening Chair Exercises

Aside from chair yoga, several other easy-to-follow exercises promote overall body strength and ease of mobility without risking injury.

Shoulder Circles

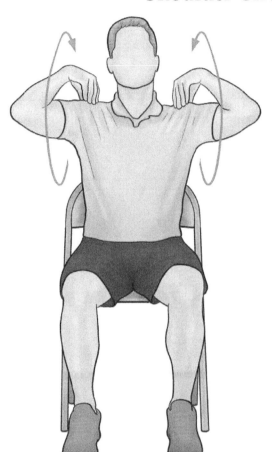

1. Sit upright in your chair and move your arms up while placing your fingertips on your shoulders.

2. Take even deep breaths in and out while slowly moving your shoulders in a circular motion forward for about 15 repetitions.

3. Pause and start reversing the circular movement for another 15 repetitions.

4. This exercise relaxes the muscles in the shoulders and avoids any possible risk of straining them.

Shoulder Circles.

Toe Taps

• Sit upright in your chair with a straight back and your feet planted firmly on the ground.

• Start bending your toes toward the ceiling and returning them back to the floor.

- If you feel this is too easy, move forward to the edge of your seat and straighten your legs.
- Make sure your heels are touching the ground at all times as you bend your toes upward and downward.

Knee Lifts

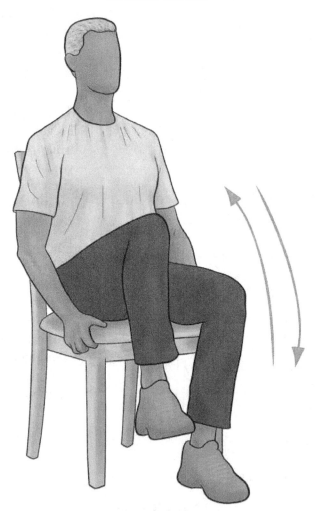

Knee Lifts.

1. Sit up straight in your chair while keeping your feet flat on the ground.
2. Inhale deeply and start to slowly raise your right leg off the floor while bending your knee in a marching position.

3. Continue to lift your leg as far as you can go without causing pain or discomfort.

4. Slowly lower your leg back to the floor and repeat the exercise with the other leg.

5. Perform 10 repetitions or as many as you can without over-exerting yourself.

As you perform these exercises, make sure to monitor your breath by taking steady, deep inhales and exhales.

These chair exercises can easily be integrated into your day-to-day activities. Set aside 5 to 15 minutes daily, whether it is in the morning once you wake up, in the afternoon, or right before you go to sleep. These practices will help relax your body and also energize you while simultaneously working on your muscle strength, overall stability, and balance. The more consistent you are, the stronger you'll feel. As you build your strength, you're also increasing your independence and improving the state of your mental health through reduced stress and anxiety levels.

Remember to pace yourself. If you rush through the exercises or ignore your pain, you may end up with an unexpected or unwanted injury.

Chapter 9: Nutrition and Hydration: Supporting Your Exercise Regime

When people think about getting in shape, they don't often consider what their nutrition should look like. You won't make that mistake because you're reading this excellent resource. In this chapter, you'll learn how to fuel your body to get the best results and recover fully from your workouts. You'll also discover the importance of staying hydrated.

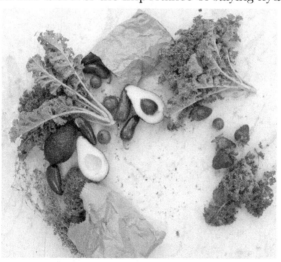

Nurture your body with the right food.
https://www.pexels.com/photo/flat-lay-photo-of-fruits-and-vegetables-1660027/

Basics of Nutrition

Many people don't know much about what's good for them to eat. What are the basics of nutrition? There are six different parts, called nutrients, that are contained in food. These tiny nutrients cannot be seen, but they are specialized to give your body energy. If you don't eat the right things, you might feel tired and weak, carrying a grumpy face that says 'do not disturb' around. So, what are these nutrients? Here's a run-through:

Carbohydrates (carbs): There are two main types of carbohydrates: simple and complex. Simple carbs, like those found in sugary drinks and white bread, provide quick but short-lived energy bursts. In contrast, complex carbs, like whole grains and vegetables, offer sustained energy and dietary fiber, which aid digestion and keep you feeling fuller for longer.

Proteins: These are the building blocks of muscles, and they help with tissue repair and growth. Choose lean protein sources like chicken, fish, beans, and lentils to avoid excess fat and saturated fat.

Healthy Fats: Not all fats perform the same functions in the body. Unsaturated fats, found in avocados, nuts, olive oil, and fatty fish, are essential for brain health, hormone production, and nutrient absorption. Make a point of reducing your intake of saturated and trans fats found in processed foods and fried items, as they can increase your risk of heart disease.

Vitamins: These micronutrients play a vital role in the various ways your body functions. Each vitamin carries with it a unique function. Vitamin D, for example, helps with bone health, while vitamin B12 supports nerve function. You can find vitamins in a variety of fruits, like avocados, oranges, lemons, and berries; vegetables, like spinach, broccoli, carrots, potatoes, and bananas; and whole grains, like rice, barley, etc.

Minerals: Minerals are the nutrients that keep things running smoothly in your body. They help your muscles work, your bones stay strong, and your heartbeat healthy and steady like a bass drum. You can find minerals in foods like meat, dairy products, and leafy green vegetables. Some common minerals include calcium, which makes your bones strong; iron, which helps your blood carry oxygen; zinc, which helps reduce the risk of diabetes; and chloride, which aids digestion and muscle function.

Water: Your body needs water to stay hydrated, regulate temperature, and get rid of waste. You can find water in fruits and vegetables, as well as in drinks like juice and milk. Drinking plenty of water every day will ensure you stay healthy and happy. Think of the times you've had the cold liquid slopping down your throat to your stomach, bringing with it that satisfying feeling that then sits in your heart. What would humans do without water?

Eating a Balanced Diet

Eating good food is important for everyone, but especially for seniors like yourself. It helps you feel strong and do things you enjoy. A good meal will also improve your physical and mental health and well-being.

Why Go for a Balanced Diet?

As people get older, staying healthy becomes even more important to them. Eating good food is like giving your body the fuel that it needs to keep it strong and active. Just like a vehicle needs the right gasoline to give its best on the highway, your body needs the right nutrients from food to feel its best. Not convinced yet? Here are a few more reasons why a balanced diet should be the order of the day.

- Your body becomes stronger: Eating healthy gives your body the building blocks it needs to keep your muscles strong, which helps you with everyday activities like walking, climbing stairs, and carrying groceries.

- You are more energetic: Good food fuels your body, giving you the energy you need to do the things you enjoy, whether it's spending time with loved ones or pursuing your hobbies.

- Your mood is usually bright and sunny: Eating balanced meals can help you feel better overall, both physically and mentally. You might feel happier, more alert, and less tired.

- It keeps your health at the top: A balanced diet helps your body fight off illnesses and stay healthy, so you don't spend time surviving instead of living and appreciating life.

Note this: Getting older means not having as much muscle as you used to, but you don't have to succumb to that fate. You need your muscles not only to look good but to feel good as you go about your day. Give your muscles a chance to show you what they are made of by feeding them eggs, Greek yogurt, avocados, nuts, lean meats like chicken and lean beef cuts, cheese, milk, beans, and fatty fish like tuna, salmon, and mackerel.

Importance of Hydration

Hydration means making sure your body has enough water to stay healthy. It's really important because water helps your body function properly. If you don't drink enough water, you can get dehydrated, which means your body doesn't have enough water to carry out its functions. When exercising, even in a seated position, you are still going to lose fluids from your body through sweating and breathing, and this can lead to dehydration. Why do you need to stay hydrated?

1. **To maintain body function:** Water is necessary for various bodily processes, including digestion, circulation, and temperature regulation. Staying hydrated can do wonders for your overall well-being.

2. **To avoid health issues:** Dehydration can increase the risk of urinary tract infections, constipation, fatigue, dizziness, and cognitive impairment in seniors. By staying properly hydrated, seniors can reduce these risks and maintain better overall health.

3. **T0 prevent dehydration:** Even if you're doing chair exercises, you still sweat and lose fluids. In order to avoid getting dehydrated, it's really important to drink water before, during, and after your workouts. Dehydration can make you feel unwell, so make sure to stay on top of your water intake.

4. **To boost your exercise performance:** As you sweat, your blood volume decreases, making it harder for your heart to pump blood throughout your body. This can lead to fatigue and muscle weakness. Drinking enough water will help you feel more energized and perform even better. When your body is properly hydrated, your muscles work better, and you can move more easily. You exercise effectively and feel less tired in the end.

5. **To prevent an increase in body temperature during exercising:** When you exercise, your body produces heat. If you're not hydrated enough, your body can't cool down properly, which can lead to overheating. You need water to regulate your body temperature and spare you from getting too hot.

6. **To speed up muscle recovery after exercise:** After chair exercises, muscles might feel sore or tired. Drinking enough

water helps speed up the recovery process. Water helps flush out toxins that build up in muscles during exercise, reducing soreness and helping seniors feel better faster.

How Do I Know My Body Needs More Water?

Not drinking enough water, which is referred to as dehydration, can leave you feeling unwell. If you aren't sure what the signs of dehydration are, answer these questions.

- Are you feeling sluggish?
- Do you have trouble thinking clearly?
- Are you having incessant headaches?
- Do your muscles feel unbearably tight or weak?
- What's the color of your urine? Is it darker than usual? (Check that when you go do your business.)
- Do you pee less often?
- Are you feeling irritable?

Strategies to Stay Hydrated

Drink plenty of water. Make a habit of drinking water throughout the day, not just when you feel thirsty. Sipping water regularly helps to maintain your hydration level.

Eat water-rich foods. Include fruits and vegetables with high water content in your diet, such as watermelons, strawberries, cucumbers, and celery.

Tame your sweet tooth and love for caffeinated beverages. Drinks like soda and coffee can actually dehydrate your body. You do not need these beverages all the time. You can opt for water or herbal tea instead.

Always check your urine color. If your urine color is dark yellow, then you are likely dehydrated. You should drink more water. The color of your urine can reveal your body's current hydration level.

Set an alarm. Who said you can't use an alarm to stay hydrated? It is more effective to set alarms and timers to remind you to drink water regularly, especially during chair exercises. The thought of it might slip your mind throughout your workout session.

Use a water bottle. Keep a water bottle handy throughout the day. Water bottles aren't made for kids alone. Adult water bottles are now available. Get one for yourself and scratch that excuse off the list. You need a water bottle to help you stay hydrated.

Now you know why good nutrition and proper hydration are necessary to improve your physical performance during and after your workouts and keep your body healthy and ready for anything. The question is: how do you make a habit of eating healthy? Where do you even begin?

Meal Planning

If you've ever struggled with disciplined eating, you need meal planning. If you already know well in advance what you're going to eat and have taken the time to prep your meals before you need them, you'll never have to battle the urge to say no to unhealthy quick fixes. When you have too many options, it's hard to make a choice. In this case, humans naturally reach for what's easy and convenient.

Use meal planning to keep you from derailing your health and fitness gains with bad food options. Proper meal planning involves knowing the recipes you'd like to prepare, creating a shopping list, getting the ingredients ahead of time from the store, and knowing when to restock so you don't fall off the wagon and resume unhealthy eating habits. It may seem like a lot of work, but you'll soon realize it isn't, especially when you notice how much time it saves you and how easy it is to stick to eating healthy meals. So, how do you plan your meals?

Make a list: Your list will keep you from getting that box of cookies or a bucket of ice cream you don't need. It keeps you from straying to the isles of the grocery store that you know you have no business being in. Now, there's no reason to have a different meal prepped for each day of the week if that feels like too much pressure. This is a new thing you're learning, so be flexible and go easy with it for starters. It's enough to have four to six meals planned out for each week since you'll probably have leftovers to enjoy the next day, dine out with friends, or enjoy takeout at least one night each week.

Get your groceries: If you're like most people, the older you get, the less eager you are to go to the store to get your groceries. The smart thing to do is set things up so you only have to go once a week, and no more than that. Even better, have your groceries sent to you by ordering online or over the phone. This way, you've removed one more hurdle between you and eating right for your health goals.

Cook your meals: Once you have all the ingredients you need, it's time to cook. If you cook every day and you're not a big fan of doing that, you may give up on meal planning altogether. So, what's the best thing to do? Pick one day when you'll cook all your meals. Sure, it'll take a considerable chunk of your time, but it's nice to know you don't have to do any cooking for the next six to seven days. Does it feel like too much work to cook it all in a day? A better option for you could be to cook in batches twice or three times a week. Don't be afraid to experiment and see what works for you.

Prepping Your Meal

At first, it may seem like meal planning and meal prepping are the same thing, but they aren't. Meal planning is about knowing what you'll eat within a fixed period and making plans for those meals. Meal prepping is about getting the components of those meals ready well before you need to cook them. This saves you cooking time, keeps you consistently eating healthy, and helps you control your portion sizes. After all, what's the point in switching to healthier meal options if you keep eating for two, right?

Here's how to prep your meals. First, make large quantities of the foods you know you'll include in each day's meal. For instance, if you always have a serving of roasted veggies and grilled chicken, you can make enough of those foods to last the week.

When you're done cooking, split your meals into portions by putting them in containers that hold enough food for one serving. It's easier to track your eating with these single-serving containers and keep yourself from giving in to the temptation of eating more than you planned. Keep the containers in the freezer or fridge, and whenever you want to eat, all you have to do is pop one in the microwave, and you have a hot meal ready to go.

Tips to Make Meal Planning and Prepping a Breeze

- The best containers are safe for use in the microwave and dishwasher.
- If you stock up on canned and frozen foods, meal prepping and cooking will be a breeze.

- Look for recipes that are not only delicious but easy to prepare. It makes no sense to feel drained at the mere thought of preparing your main ingredients, let alone putting them together.
- If you cut up your ingredients ahead of time, your future self will thank you for being so considerate. Even better – buy your groceries pre-cut.
- If there are ingredients you'll always have to cut, do the cutting at once before you need them.
- As soon as you're back from the store, properly wash your fruits and veggies using three parts water to one part white distilled vinegar. Let the fresh ingredients sit in the solution for at least three minutes, rinse them with plain water, pat them dry, and then store them in their respective compartments in the fridge.
- Change things up now and then so you're not bored of your meals.
- When you really can't find it in you to cook, ask for help from the people you live with. There's no reason why you have to go it alone if you are blessed with family and friends around you.

Recipes

Now that you know how to plan and prep your meals, you could use a few delicious recipes that are easy to prepare and fuel your body with good energy.

Tomato Tart

Would you like a healthy dose of vitamin C to keep your body strong and your immune system active as it should be? Then, this is a great recipe to try.

Ingredients:
- 1 thawed sheet of frozen puff pastry
- 1 onion (sliced thin)
- 1 tablespoon chopped fresh herbs (basil, oregano, etc.) Or 1 tablespoon of your favorite Italian seasoning
- 1 cup of cheese (feta, parmesan, mozzarella, blue cheese, or any other kind you prefer)
- 2 large tomatoes (make it three if you'd love a little more red)

- 1 teaspoon olive oil
- Salt or salt replacement (to taste)
- Pepper (to taste)

Instructions:

1. Whip out your baking sheet and line it with nonstick aluminum foil or parchment paper. Please don't use wax paper.
2. Preheat your oven. You want it to be at 425 F.
3. Get your puff pastry and give it a good stretch on the lined sheet.
4. Grab a fork. Using the prongs, poke some holes along the bottom of the pastry.
5. Put a skillet on the stove over medium heat. Add your olive oil to it.
6. Throw the onions into the skillet and keep stirring while you saute them until they're nice and soft. This shouldn't take longer than five minutes.
7. Once your onions are ready, spread them over the pastry dough.
8. Slice your tomatoes thinly and top the onions with them. Don't let the slices overlap.
9. Sprinkle your cheese over the tomatoes, then add half of the herbs or Italian seasoning.
10. Season the top with salt and pepper. Don't use too much salt, and if you're not supposed to have too much sodium, please use your salt replacement instead.
11. Sprinkle as much pepper as you like (or skip the pepper if you don't care for the burn.
12. Pop the baking sheet into the oven and let your tart bake for the next 25 minutes. When it's ready, the crust should have a nice golden color.
13. Using mittens, remove your tart from the oven and sprinkle the rest of your herbs on top. Then, cut the tart into little squares and enjoy your meal.

Salmon and Veggies

The lovely thing about this recipe is that all you need is one pan. It's so easy to prepare, and your heart will thank you for the omega-3 fatty acids you're feeding it. Thanks to the vitamin B from this meal, you'll also have more energy. If you're tired of salmon or want to try something else, you could use any other flaky fish. Trout or tilapia will work for this recipe as well.

Ingredients:

- ½ onion (in wedges)
- 1 zucchini or squash (in rounds)
- 1 bell pepper (sliced)
- 1 cup grape or cherry tomatoes
- 1 teaspoon Cajun seasoning (you can replace this with a different fish seasoning blend if you prefer)
- 3 tablespoons olive oil
- 2 or 3 salmon fillets (make it 4 ounces each)
- 1 lemon (optional)

Instructions:

1. Preheat your oven to 450 F.
2. Get your trusty baking sheet and line it with aluminum foil or parchment paper. If you don't have either, grease your sheet with some vegetable oil.
3. Grab a large bowl and throw in all your veggies.
4. Add your seasoning and 2 tablespoons of oil to the veggie bowl. Save the third tablespoon for later.
5. Spread your veggies out on the sheet so it's a nice, even layer.
6. Place the salmon fillets between the veggies. Check to be sure you have the skin side down.
7. With the last tablespoon of olive oil, brush the salmon.
8. Set two thin lemon slices on each of the fillets.
9. Pop the baking sheet into the oven and let it all roast for 12 to 15 minutes. You'll know it's ready when the salmon looks opaque and flakes easily.
10. Each serving should have one salmon fillet, along with the roasted veggies. Bon Appetit.

Chicken and Berry Salad

If you want a plate that pops with color and protein to give you strong muscles, you'll love this recipe. It's an excellent meal to put together when you have leftover chicken. The antioxidants from the berries are another benefit of having this meal.

Ingredients:

- Torn salad greens (spinach works, too)
- ½ cup celery (chopped)
- ½ cup fresh peas (you can use frozen peas instead as long as they're thawed)
- 1 teaspoon sugar
- ¼ cup olive oil mayonnaise (regular mayo is okay, but know it's high in cholesterol)
- ½ teaspoon tarragon (dried)
- 1 cup fresh blueberries (whole) Or strawberries (quartered)
- 1 ½ cups leftover chicken (shredded or chopped)

Instructions:

1. Grab a bowl and whisk your olive oil mayo, sugar, and dried tarragon together in it.
2. Toss the chicken, peas, celery, and berries into the bowl.
3. Give the ingredients in your bowl a thorough stir, so they combine evenly.
4. Serve your spinach or salad greens on a plate, then top the greens with your chicken and berry salad for a healthy, delicious, and filling meal.

Tuna Veggie Casserole

This meal is a good one to prepare when you're not in the mood for fancy cooking but want to give your body something nutritious.

Ingredients:

- 1 cup cheddar cheese (shredded)
- 1 bag whole wheat egg noodles (12 ounces)
- 2 cans cream of mushroom soup (10 ¾ ounces each)

- ½ cup milk
- 2 cans tuna (drained, 5 ounces each)
- 2 cups frozen veggies (try carrots, peas, broccoli, or a combo)
- 8 buttery crackers (Ritz or something like it)
- Salt or salt replacement (to taste)
- Pepper (to taste, optional)

Instructions:

1. Get your oven ready by preheating it to 350 F.
2. Find your 3-quart casserole dish. Don't have one? Use a baking pan that's 13 inches by 9 inches. Grease the dish or pan.
3. Following the instructions on the package, cook your whole wheat noodles. When you're done, drain them so there's no liquid left.
4. Mix the cheese, milk, veggies, mushroom soup, and tuna with your noodles.
5. Season the mix with salt and pepper.
6. Scoop this mix onto your greased dish or pan.
7. Crush the crackers into little chunks, and then spread them evenly on top of your casserole. If you want extra cheese – no one's stopping you. Go for it.
8. Pop your casserole in the oven and let it sit for the next 20 minutes. You'll know it's ready when it's a lovely golden color, barely starting to go brown. Serve and enjoy this delicious meal while it's warm.

Bean Salad

If you want something easy, try this recipe on for size.

Ingredients:

- ⅓ cup olive oil
- ½ cup white sugar (use ¼ cup honey to make it healthier)
- ⅔ cup white vinegar or apple cider vinegar
- 1 thinly sliced white onion (yellow onion also works)
- 1 can chickpeas (15 ounces, drained and rinsed)
- 1 can kidney beans (15 ounces, drained and rinsed)
- 1 can green beans (15 ounces, drained and rinsed)

- 1 can wax beans (15 ounces, drained and rinsed)
- Salt (to taste)
- Pepper (to taste)

Instructions:

1. Get the largest Tupperware container or bowl you have. Throw all your ingredients in it.
2. Mix all the ingredients thoroughly.
3. Pop it in the refrigerator and let it sit overnight or for some hours so it can marinate.
4. Serve as a topping for your green salads or as a side when you're enjoying some grilled chicken.

These are just a few of the amazing recipes you could try. Don't be afraid to get creative with them, and you'll find that eating healthy isn't a chore. When your body shows you the results of your food choices and your decision to stay properly hydrated, you'll never want to stop living and treating yourself right.

When you eat healthy foods and drink enough water, it gives you the energy and strength you need to do your exercises well. Plus, it helps your muscles and joints work better, so you can move around more easily. When you have good nutrition and hydration, you're more likely to feel good during and after your exercises. It also helps your body recover faster, so you can keep exercising regularly without feeling tired or sore all the time. So, don't joke with your tummy. Start eating right today and drink plenty of water to help you stay active and feel your best as you do these chair exercises.

Chapter 10: Making It a Lifestyle: Integrating Chair Exercises into Daily Life

After reading this chapter, you'll understand what habits are and how they can transform your life for the better. You'll find out why habits are the key to shaping your life and working closer toward your goals, understanding how they're better than inspiration and motivation. You'll also understand the importance of chair exercises and learn how sitting for prolonged periods can hinder your posture and weaken pivotal muscles. This chapter offers helpful tips and micro-exercises for maintaining your posture and engaging your core muscles in your daily life. It also provides a few simple yet effective breathing techniques that can enhance the health of your lungs and your overall well-being.

What Are Habits?

People pick up numerous habits from the day they set foot into the world, whether they're aware of doing them or not. Once you wake up, you automatically make your way to the restroom to brush your teeth. When you step into the shower, you might immediately reach for the shampoo bottle, even if it's not hair-wash day. When you engage in habits, your brain somewhat goes into autopilot. Your brain and body are already aware of what they need to do, requiring less conscious effort, focus, and engagement on your part. This allows you to cater to your needs and do some of your tasks more efficiently throughout the day.

Habits become so deeply ingrained into your system that even the most harmful ones, such as smoking, for instance, are very challenging to break. Doing something beneficial so often that it becomes a habit can transform your life. It can boost your self-esteem and confidence because it helps you realize that you're powerful enough to make substantial changes in your life.

The Importance of Developing Healthy Habits

- **They Make You Feel Less Overwhelmed**

    Developing healthy habits helps you realize that you're capable of becoming the person you want to be. Say you want to finish reading a certain book. You'd feel less overwhelmed if you got into the habit of reading a few pages every day or designating the time before you go to bed to read. When you find that you've managed to complete this book and take on other reading challenges, you'll feel more motivated to stick to this behavior.

- **They Lower Stress and Anxiety Levels**

    Developing rewarding habits can lower your stress and anxiety because they make your life feel more structured and organized. For instance, if you make it a habit to prepare your meals for the entire week during the weekend, you'll be able to stick to your healthy eating goals if you have no time to prepare nutritious meals throughout the week.

- **They Improve the Quality of Your Life**

    Your habits largely shape who you are because they are activities that you do several times a day without thinking about them. They become imprinted in your psyche, and going a while without them can feel very unusual. They have a profound effect on the quality of your life. Understanding the impact that habits have on your life and well-being encourages you to engage in more beneficial behaviors and actively work toward breaking unhealthy ones. By taking control of your habits, you can live a life that aligns with your goals, aspirations, beliefs, and values.

- **They Can Be Altered**

    One great thing about habits is that they can be altered. You don't have to live with them forever. While changing bad habits can be challenging, especially if you've stuck with them for years, these changes are still possible with enough dedication. The key is to break down the changes that you need to make in order to change certain habits into manageable steps. Create milestones that will help you become the person you want to be.

- **They Lead You Closer Toward Your Goals**

Some of the greatest companies in the world, like Amazon, Apple, Dell, Google, Microsoft, and Walt Disney and Co., were all built-in garages. They didn't become giants overnight. They would rather spend years refining their products or changing them altogether and upscaling their strategies. Their founders went through numerous phases of trial and error – continuously searching for the best way to improve their businesses. If these world-renowned companies started this small once and needed decades to get where they are today, you, too, can't achieve your goals overnight.

Imagine you want to run a marathon but have never had any proper training for it. You can't just buy a new pair of running shoes and go for it, right? To run a marathon, you need to gradually build up your capabilities mile by mile. You also need to eat a more balanced, healthier diet that helps strengthen your muscles and gives you more energy. Whenever you want to achieve a goal, regardless of how big or small it is, you need to determine the habits you need to acquire, the habits you need to strengthen, and the ones you need to let go of to ensure that you're headed in the right direction.

- **They Are More Effective Than Motivation**

Many people believe that motivation is the key to success. However, if you think about it, you'll find that it's hard to always stay motivated. Everyone has bad days or gets distracted at times. It's very hard to power through rough patches in life, let alone stay driven and inspired. If you're very busy, the last thing you might think about is spending time with your family or making sure you stay healthy. However, if these behaviors become habits, you'll do them without thinking. You'll no longer have to garner every ounce of motivation to get things done. Habits are easier and more effective than motivation.

The Importance of Chair Exercises

Physical exercise is just as important, if not more so, to older individuals as it is to younger people. Maintaining your mobility and range of motion is crucial as you age because it allows you to prevent certain age-related diseases, improve cardiovascular health, enhance cognitive function, and maintain muscle mass and bone density. That said, it's nearly impossible to move freely without putting strain on your body as you get older. This is where chair exercises can come in handy. Chair exercises offer the same benefits as regular workouts for individuals who struggle to maintain their balance or have limited mobility and range of motion.

Making chair exercises a habit and incorporating them into your daily routine can increase your blood flow, reduce your risk of falling, strengthen your muscles, and boost joint health. Better blood flow can improve your cardiovascular health because it ensures that oxygen and nutrients are delivered to all your organs. Several chair exercises focus on strengthening certain muscle groups, enhancing your balance and stability, and lowering your risk of falling. Chair exercises are gentle, low-impact, and effective. They gradually build up your flexibility and reduce stiffness in your joints. Chair exercises encourage your joints to navigate their entire range of motion, which can allow you to prevent or alleviate medical conditions like arthritis.

The older you get, the more likely you are to spend a lot of time sitting. Staying seated for long periods can cause noticeable changes in your posture. It trains your pelvis to tilt backward. Over time, your hips become weaker and are no longer able to support your upper body. Sitting, as opposed to walking, doesn't engage your core and glute muscles, which are necessary for supporting the spine.

When all these bones and muscles fail to do their jobs effectively, the spine transforms from looking like an S to a C-like shape. This keeps you from standing up straight and causes you to develop a slouched posture. If you can't walk around and work out as you used to, you might as well do chair exercises. They can help you maintain your natural posture and keep the situation from deteriorating. These workouts are highly focused on helping you maintain your posture. They train you to sit up tall and teach you to align your ears, shoulders, and hips. They also actively engage your core and glute muscles to ensure that your spine stays supported.

Exercises for Improving Posture

Belly Exercise

Sit upright and keep your back as straight as possible. Draw a deep breath as you gradually tighten your belly. Imagine that you're trying to bring your belly button to your spine. As you do so, avoid tilting your head forward. Keep your neck straight while slightly tucking in your chin. Imagine that a string is pulling you from the top of your head toward the sky. After you achieve the right posture, focus on breathing deeply. Inhale from your belly rather than from your chest. Notice your belly expanding, followed by your chest. Hold this position for a few seconds as you notice how your body feels. Bring your attention to how your ears, shoulders, and hips are aligned, using these simple exercises as a foundation for the following chair exercises.

Shoulder Exercise

Pick this exercise up where the belly exercise left your posture. As you sit tall, bring your shoulders up toward your ears, then gently roll them to the front. Bring them from the front down, then rotate them back to their initial position, then up again. Then, re-do them in the other direction. After you bring your shoulders up, roll them to the back, bring them from the back downward, then rotate them forward to their initial centered position, then up again. Do this exercise ten times, alternating between directions.

Knee Exercises

Start this exercise with your ears, shoulders, and hips aligned. Slowly lift your right knee, bringing it up toward your chest, then return it back to where it was. Gently do the same with your other knee. Start by doing this exercise 10 times, alternating between knees. Gradually build up your capacity over time. It's okay if you can only endure less than 10 counts the first time. Do your best, and try to do more counts as you progress. This exercise will strengthen your belly, core, and quad muscles.

When you're done with this exercise, scoot forward to the edge of the chair. Preferably, sit in an armchair to hold on to the armrest for support. If it's not available, hold on to the edges of the chair, but make sure you feel balanced before starting this exercise. When you're ready, lift your right leg up, extending the calf. Try your best to create a straight line from the edge of the chair. Keep your toes facing upward toward the ceiling. Your knees can slightly bend so they're not locked. Hold for a few seconds before gently bringing your leg back to the starting position. Do the same with your other leg and continue alternating for 10 counts or for as long as you're able to.

Upper-Body Exercises

Picking up where you left off, at the edge of the chair, stretch both your arms forward. Practice staying balanced in this position before you progress further into this exercise. When you're ready, slightly bend your elbows while aligning them with your centerline. Your thumb should be facing toward the ceiling. Pull your elbows as far back as you can, making sure that your shoulders and arms are squeezed in. Your arms shouldn't be positioned far away from your body. Do this exercise for 10 counts or for as long as you can endure.

Tips for Improving Your Posture

- Exercising regularly will help you enhance your posture. Doing as little as 30 minutes of chair exercises or any other low-impact workout a day can help you improve your range of motion and keep you active. This will also enhance your overall health and well-being.

- The gentle exercises mentioned throughout this book will help you strengthen your back and belly muscles. They are also designed to help you correct your posture and strengthen your core muscles. Ten minutes of stretching exercises a day also helps.

- Avoid crossing your legs when you're sitting down. Depending on which leg you're used to crossing over, this position can overstretch one side of your leg muscles. When this happens, the alignment of your spine will change.

- Practice standing tall. Keep your spine straight and focus on maintaining the natural resting position of your shoulders. Many people tend to shrug their shoulders when they're tense or stressed. Tighten your stomach muscles gently to engage your core muscles and support your spine. Tightening shouldn't feel uncomfortable but rather like an activation of these muscles.

- While it might seem comfortable or natural, avoid sitting on very soft or low-seated chairs or sofas for too long.

- If you can easily stand back up without help, lie down on the ground for a couple of minutes once a day. Keep your body flat, pressed to the floor, without using cushions or blankets to support it. Relax, allowing your body to adjust to its natural resting position. This will allow it to recorrect its posture over time.

- When going out, pick out the right pair of shoes. Make sure that they're flat and correctly fitted — neither too loose nor too tight. Wearing the right shoes will ensure that your weight is distributed evenly.

- When lifting heavy items, make sure that you're lifting them up using your hips, thighs, and knees. Don't lift with your back.

- Move your head every day to loosen tight neck muscles. Tightness can often prevent good body posture. Take a few minutes to gently move your head around in small circles, front to back and side to side.

- When you're sleeping, rest your head on one firm support pillow to avoid developing neck pains or conditions.

- The best positions for maintaining spine posture are lying on your side with your knees bent and a pillow between your legs or on your back with a pillow under your knees.

Engaging Your Core

You use your core muscles in nearly everything you do, so engaging and strengthening them is crucial. How you actively engage your core depends on the activity you're doing. The first step, however, is understanding how it feels to engage them and knowing which muscles are in use. Many people confuse engaging the core with sucking in the belly, not understanding that the latter is counter-productive. Sucking in your belly can weaken your core muscles over time. It puts pressure on your back and neck, makes breathing hard, and is very uncomfortable to endure.

This exercise will help you understand how your body should feel when you're engaging your core in your daily life:

Inhale, drawing in a deep breath from your diaphragm. Exhale as you tighten your belly, bringing in your belly button toward your spine. Tighten further until you feel that the muscles in your lower back, as well as those in the front and sides of your core, are engaged. You shouldn't be in pain as you do this. Hold this position for a few seconds before releasing. Do this a few times, ensuring that you give your muscles enough time to relax in between to avoid fatiguing them.

Breathing Techniques

The following are a few simple breathing techniques that can enhance the function of your lungs and improve your health:

Complete Breathing

Most people don't notice that they're not breathing as thoroughly as they should. This exercise ensures that your breaths are complete and that oxygen effectively reaches different parts of your body. It engages your upper chest, diaphragm, and lower ribcage to help you achieve deep breaths.

To practice this technique, you need to sit up straight, aligning your ears, shoulders, and hips. Close your eyes, exhale, and then inhale, allowing all your stomach muscles to relax. As you draw in your breath, feel your belly expanding, filling up with air. Keep breathing until your chest also expands as it accommodates the air. Hold for a few seconds before exhaling slowly. Release every last breath, feeling the air exit your lungs and your stomach tightening slightly. Do this for a few minutes every day.

Humming Breathing

As you can deduce from its name, this exercise involves humming, particularly when you exhale. It stimulates your cognitive functions and enhances your physical health. To do this exercise, you need to follow the instructions provided for complete breathing. The only twist is that you hum as you exhale and release all the air from your chest and belly. Tighten your belly muscles as you hum, and then relax. Repeat this exercise a couple of times.

Diaphragmatic Breathing

This exercise will help you relax and remove tension from your body. It also engages your diaphragm to ensure more thorough breathing. Lie on your back, placing one hand on your stomach and the other right below it on your navel. Bring your attention to your diaphragm, ensuring that you draw your breaths from it. You'll know that you're doing this technique right when you see the hand on your navel rise before the other one does.

Now that you've read the final chapter of this book, you are encouraged to incorporate chair exercises into your daily routine. Practicing chair exercises is a journey toward enhancing your overall well-being. These techniques can transform your mental, emotional, and physical health.

Conclusion

Chair yoga isn't just your run-of-the-mill fitness program – it's a game-changer. Whether you're dealing with physical limitations like multiple sclerosis, cardiovascular issues, or pulmonary disease, chair yoga is your ticket to an enjoyable and approachable workout routine. Don't let the word "chair" fool you – this practice can be just as challenging as traditional yoga. The thing is, no matter your fitness level or health condition, you can find motivation and a sense of accomplishment through physical activity.

To do this, there's no need to contort yourself into impossible positions or endure grueling workouts. Chair yoga meets you where you are, whether you're a beginner or are used to exercising, and it offers a gentle yet effective path to wellness. Age is just a number in the world of chair yoga. Whether you're a seasoned yogi or a complete newbie, you can reap the benefits of this practice. Even if you're seated for the entire session or using the chair for support, you're still in for a transformative experience.

Now, let's debunk a myth – chair yoga isn't just for seniors. It's for anyone looking to build confidence, improve their physical and emotional well-being, and try something new. Plus, with props like chairs in the mix, the possibilities for mindful movement are endless. Throughout this book, you've explored a variety of poses and techniques designed specifically for seniors, addressing common concerns like mobility, back pain, posture, and balance. But beyond the physical benefits, chair yoga offers something deeper – a sense of peace, relaxation, and connection with your body.

By incorporating simple breathing exercises and mindful movements into your daily routine, you'll begin to notice a shift - tension melting away, muscles relaxing, and a newfound sense of ease in your body and mind. No longer will you have to feel limited by age or physical condition. With chair yoga, the possibilities are endless, and the journey is yours to explore. And, for all you beginners out there, listen up: chair yoga poses are the perfect starting point for your practice. You'll improve your coordination, balance, and range of motion, all while maintaining proper posture and alignment.

So, if you're looking for a hobby that'll tick all the boxes - physical, emotional, and everything in between - look no further than yoga. And remember, the journey starts right here, right now, in your very own chair. So, roll out that yoga mat (or grab your favorite chair), take a deep breath, and continue on this beautiful journey.

Here's another book by Scott Hamrick that you might like

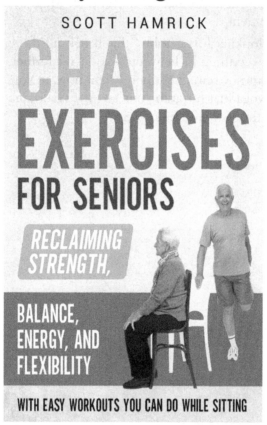

Free Bonuses from Scott Hamrick available for limited time

Hi seniors!

My name is Scott Hamrick, and first off, I want to THANK YOU for reading my book.

Now you have a chance to join my exclusive "workout for seniors" email list so you can get the ebook below for free as well as the potential to get more ebooks for seniors for free! Simply click the link below to join.

P.S. Remember that it's 100% free to join the list.

Access your free bonuses here

https://livetolearn.lpages.co/chair-exercises-for-seniors-28-day-paperback/

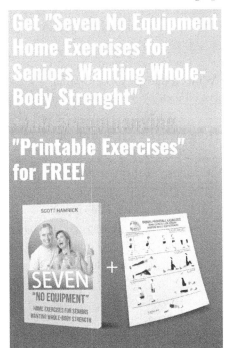

Or, Scan the QR code!

References

6 reasons why chair-based exercise is good for you. (n.d.). LiveWell Dorset. https://www.livewelldorset.co.uk/faq/get-active/6-reasons-why-chair-based-exercise-is-good-for-you/

7 Benefits of Improved Posture at Work + Exercises to Help. (2020, August 24). University of St. Augustine for Health Sciences. https://www.usa.edu/blog/how-to-improve-posture/

13 Benefits of Strength Training for People Older Than 50. (n.d.). Human Kinetics Canada. https://canada.humankinetics.com/blogs/articles/13-benefits-of-strength-training-for-people-older-than-50

Asher, A. (n.d.). How to Relieve Back Pain With Achieving Good Spinal Alignment. Verywell Health. https://www.verywellhealth.com/posture-and-alignment-296665

Benefits of Chair Exercises for Seniors. (2021, September 21). CareLink. https://www.carelink.org/benefits-of-chair-exercises-for-seniors/

Bowen, V. (2023). Maintaining Flexibility With Aging. Arthritis and Rheumatism Associates, P.C. https://arapc.com/maintaining-flexibility-with-aging/

British Heart Foundation. (2019). 5 more easy chair exercises. Bhf.org.uk. https://www.bhf.org.uk/informationsupport/heart-matters-magazine/activity/chair-based-exercises/5-more-chair-based-exercises

CDC. (2021, February 17). How much physical activity do older adults need? | Physical Activity | CDC. Www.cdc.gov. https://www.cdc.gov/physicalactivity/basics/older_adults/index.htm

Chair Based Exercise. (n.d.). Faversham & Sittingbourne. https://www.ageuk.org.uk/favershamandsittingbourne/our-services/centre-based-activities/chair-based-exercise/

Chair exercises are beneficial for older adults - Oklahoma State University. (2021, December 22). Extension.okstate.edu. https://extension.okstate.edu/articles/2021/chair-exercises.html

Cleveland Clinic. (2019, November 19). Skeletal System. Cleveland Clinic. https://my.clevelandclinic.org/health/body/21048-skeletal-system

Cleveland Clinic. (2022, June 3). Sarcopenia (Muscle Loss): Symptoms & Causes. Cleveland Clinic. https://my.clevelandclinic.org/health/diseases/23167-sarcopenia

Cristol, H. (2021, March 26). How Posture Changes as You Get Older. WebMD. https://www.webmd.com/healthy-aging/features/posture-changes-older-adults

Davda, R. (n.d.). 15 In-Chair Exercises to Keep You Moving | Garage Gym Reviews. In-Chair Exercises for Seniors: Get Stronger with These 15 Movements. https://www.garagegymreviews.com/in-chair-exercises

Davenport, S. (2022, November 15). How and why to try chair exercises. Www.medicalnewstoday.com. https://www.medicalnewstoday.com/articles/how-and-why-to-try-chair-exercises#tips-for-beginners

Deguara, C. (2023, December 28). How And Why To Try Chair Exercises! Brio Leisure. https://www.brioleisure.org/blog/how-and-why-to-try-chair-exercises

E. Budson, A. (2021, December 2). How to stay strong and coordinated as you age. Harvard Health. https://www.health.harvard.edu/blog/how-to-stay-strong-and-coordinated-as-you-age-202112022651

Eicher, A. (2017, October 11). Exercise: The Value of Slow and Controlled Movements. Www.linkedin.com. https://www.linkedin.com/pulse/exercise-value-slow-controlled-movements-aubrey-eicher/

Fitness - A Guide to Chair Exercises. (2022, March 22). 5 Bridges Health & Fitness. https://5bridgeshealthandfitness.com/blog/a-guide-to-chair-exercises/

Furtado, G. E., Carvalho, H. M., Loureiro, M., Patrício, M., Uba-Chupel, M., Colado, J. C., Hogervorst, E., Ferreira, J. P., & Teixeira, A. M. (2020). Chair-based exercise programs in institutionalized older women: Salivary steroid hormones, disabilities, and frailty changes. Experimental Gerontology, 130, 110790. https://doi.org/10.1016/j.exger.2019.110790

Harvard Health. (2021, July 20). Endorphins: The brain's natural pain reliever. Harvard Health. https://www.health.harvard.edu/mind-and-mood/endorphins-the-brains-natural-pain-reliever

How To Improve Balance For Seniors by Doing Simple Moves. (n.d.). Https://Restorativestrength.com/. https://restorativestrength.com/how-to-improve-your-balance-exercises/

Importance of Good Posture for Seniors. (2021, September 15). Franciscan Ministries. https://franciscanministries.org/blog/importance-of-posture-for-seniors-2/

Mary Anne Dunkin. (2022, November 20). Sarcopenia With Aging. WebMD. https://www.webmd.com/healthy-aging/sarcopenia-with-aging

McCoy, J. (n.d.). What Trainers Really Mean When They Tell You to "Engage Your Core." Health. https://www.health.com/fitness/how-to-engage-your-core

Mill, M. (2020, January 28). 18 Chair Exercises for Seniors & How to Get Started. Vive Health. https://www.vivehealth.com/blogs/resources/chair-exercises-for-seniors

NHS. (2018, April 30). Sitting exercises. Nhs.uk. https://www.nhs.uk/live-well/exercise/sitting-exercises/

Older Adults and Balance Problems. (n.d.). National Institute on Aging. https://www.nia.nih.gov/health/falls-and-falls-prevention/older-adults-and-balance-problems#symptoms

Proper Body Alignment. (n.d.). Bone Health & Osteoporosis Foundation. https://www.bonehealthandosteoporosis.org/patients/treatment/exercisesafe-movement/proper-body-alignment/

Purvi Kalra. (2023, August 14). Strength training for seniors: Here's why this exercise is important for older adults. Healthshots. https://www.healthshots.com/fitness/muscle-gain/strength-training-for-seniors/

Robinson, K. R., Masud, T., & Hawley-Hague, H. (2016). Instructors' Perceptions of Mostly Seated Exercise Classes: Exploring the Concept of Chair Based Exercise. BioMed Research International, 2016, 1–8. https://doi.org/10.1155/2016/3241873

Services, D. of H. & H. (n.d.). Physical activity for seniors. www.betterhealth.vic.gov.au. https://www.betterhealth.vic.gov.au/health/healthyliving/physical-activity-for-seniors#physical-decline-of-older-age

Smiley, K. (2023, July 28). Improve Balance and Stability with Chair Exercises for Chronic Conditions. Smileys Points. https://smileyspoints.com/improve-balance-and-stability-with-chair-exercises-for-chronic-conditions/#improve-stability

Trudi's TEN for Fitness Professionals: 10 Reasons Why Chair-Based Exercise is Great. (n.d.). Www.thirdagefitness.com.au. https://www.thirdagefitness.com.au/pages/trudis-ten-for-professionals-10-reasons-why-we-love-chair-based-exercise

Why Proper Posture Is Imperative For Seniors - Senior Living & Nursing Homes In Indiana | ASC. (2016, January 7). Www.asccare.com. https://www.asccare.com/why-proper-posture-is-imperative-for-seniors/

Yoshimura, Y., Wakabayashi, H., Nagano, F., Bise, T., Shimazu, S., & Shiraishi, A. (2020). Chair-stand exercise improves post-stroke dysphagia. Geriatrics & Gerontology International, 20(10), 885–891. https://doi.org/10.1111/ggi.13998

Your questions about chair workouts answered – Age Bold. (n.d.). Agebold.com. https://agebold.com/blog/5-top-seated-workout-questions-and-3-simple-at-home-seated-exercises/

zpthemetest. (2020, May 1). 5 Reasons to Lift with Slow and Controlled Movements. Cannon Fitness and Performance. https://cannonfitnessandperformance.com/lift-slow-controlled-movements/

Laura Williams. (2020). 11 Accessible Chair Exercises for Older Adults. Verywell Fit. https://www.verywellfit.com/chair-exercises-for-seniors-4161267

14 Seated & Chair Exercises For Seniors. (n.d.). Lifeline. https://www.lifeline.ca/en/resources/chair-exercises-for-seniors/

Biswas, C. (2021, October 11). 15 Easy And Effective Chair Exercises For Seniors. STYLECRAZE. https://www.stylecraze.com/articles/chair-exercises-for-seniors/

Confidence and positive attitude help older adults stick with exercise. (n.d.). Human Kinetics. https://us.humankinetics.com/blogs/excerpt/confidence-and-positive-attitude-help-older-adults-stick-with-exercise

Cronkleton, E. (2019, April 9). 10 Breathing Exercises to Try: For Stress, Training, and Lung Capacity. Healthline. https://www.healthline.com/health/breathing-exercise#resonant-

Davda, R. (n.d.). 15 In-Chair Exercises to Keep You Moving | Garage Gym Reviews. In-Chair Exercises for Seniors: Get Stronger with These 15 Movements. https://garagegymreviews.com/in-chair-exercises

HIA Guest. (2020, June 9). Keep Moving to Prevent Major Mobility Disability > Health in Aging Blog > Health in Aging. Keep Moving to Prevent Major Mobility Disability. https://www.healthinaging.org/blog/keep-moving-to-prevent-major-mobility-disability/

Improving your mobility. (2022, December 7). Harvard Health. https://www.health.harvard.edu/exercise-and-fitness/improving-your-mobility

ISSA. (2022, July 13). 5 Ways Exercise Builds Self-Confidence—Plus Real Inspiration | ISSA. Www.issaonline.com. https://www.issaonline.com/blog/post/jessenia-gallegos-breaking-free-and-finding-sanctuary-in-fitness

Jennifer Boidy. (2018, October 29). What Happens to Your Body When You Stop Working Out? - InBody USA. InBody USA. https://inbodyusa.com/blogs/inbodyblog/what-happens-when-you-stop-working-out/

Kirkova, D. (2015, October 23). Here's what happens to your body when you stop exercising. Metro. https://metro.co.uk/2015/10/23/what-happens-to-your-body-when-you-stop-exercising-5456530/

Leonard, J. (n.d.). Building muscle with exercise: How muscle builds, routines, and diet. Www.medicalnewstoday.com. https://www.medicalnewstoday.com/articles/319151#rest-and-muscle-growth

Leyva, J. (2013, September 17). How Do Muscles Grow? The Science of Muscle Growth. BuiltLean. https://www.builtlean.com/muscles-grow/

Lindberg, S. (2022, January 10). 9 Total-Body Exercises You Can Do With Just a Chair. SELF. https://www.self.com/gallery/chair-exercises

Living, A. S. S. (n.d.). 9 Activities for Seniors That Can Improve Self-Confidence | All Seasons Senior Living. 9 Activities for Seniors That Can Improve Self-Confidence. https://allseasonsseniorliving.com/9-activities-for-seniors-that-can-improve-self-confidence/

Mayo Clinic. (2021, October 8). 7 great reasons why exercise matters. Mayo Clinic; Mayo Foundation for Medical Education and Research. https://www.mayoclinic.org/healthy-lifestyle/fitness/in-depth/exercise/art-20048389

Semeco, A. (2017, February 10). Exercise: The Top 10 Benefits of Regular Physical Activity. Healthline. https://www.healthline.com/nutrition/10-benefits-of-exercise#chronic-disease

seo_team. (2022, December 14). Senior Chair Exercises | Seasons Retirements. Seasons Retirement Communities. https://seasonsretirement.com/10-senior-chair-exercises/

Sherrell, Z. (2023, May 26). Chair Exercises: 13 Best Workouts for Whole Body. Greatist. https://greatist.com/fitness/chair-exercises#chair-squats

Physical activity - how to get active when you are busy - Better Health Channel. (n.d.). Www.betterhealth.vic.gov.au. https://www.betterhealth.vic.gov.au/health/healthyliving/Physical-activity-how-to-get-active-when-you-are-busy#how-to-fit-activity-into-your-life

Iliades, Chris. "The Benefits of Strength and Weight Training | Everyday Health." EverydayHealth.com, 30 Jan. 2018, www.everydayhealth.com/fitness/add-strength-training-to-your-workout.aspx.

Integrated Rehabilitation Services. "Benefits of Increasing Upper Body Strength | Integrated Rehab." Integrated Rehabilitation Services, 15 Apr. 2021, integrehab.com/blog/strength-and-conditioning/upper-body-strength/.

Waehner, Paige. "Total Body Strength Workout for Seniors Builds Stability." Verywell Fit, 5 June 2023, www.verywellfit.com/total-body-strength-workout-for-seniors-1230958.

Wenndt, Lindsay. "The 9 Chair Exercises Seniors Can Do for Better Health and Mobility." GoodRx, GoodRx, 5 Oct. 2022, www.goodrx.com/well-being/movement-exercise/20-chair-exercises-for-seniors.

Zorzan, Nadia. "Best Chair Exercises for Seniors: Safe and Easy Workouts." Www.medicalnewstoday.com, 31 Oct. 2022, www.medicalnewstoday.com/articles/chair-exercises-for-seniors.

California Mobility. "21 Chair Exercises for Seniors: Complete Visual Guide - California Mobility." California Mobility, 14 Dec. 2018, californiamobility.com/21-chair-exercises-for-seniors-visual-guide/.

Davenport, Suzy. "How and Why to Try Chair Exercises." Www.medicalnewstoday.com, 15 Nov. 2022, www.medicalnewstoday.com/articles/how-and-why-to-try-chair-exercises.

https://www.facebook.com/verywell. "11 Accessible Chair Exercises for Older Adults." Verywell Fit, 2020, www.verywellfit.com/chair-exercises-for-seniors-4161267.

Lindberg, Sara. "Seated and Standing Chair Exercises for Seniors." Healthline, 10 Mar. 2020, www.healthline.com/health/chair-exercises-for-seniors.

8 core exercises for seniors (pictures included). (2022, February 28). Lifeline. https://www.lifeline.ca/en/resources/core-exercises-for-seniors/

Chris Freytag, C. P. T. (2024, February 9). 8 best core exercises for seniors to build strength. Get Healthy U | Chris Freytag; Get Healthy U. https://gethealthyu.com/best-core-exercises-for-seniors/

Christian. (2023, December 12). 5 easy seated abdominal exercises to strengthen your core. Kustom Kit Gym Equipment; Christian. https://kustomkitgymequipment.com/blogs/news/seated-abdominal-exercises/

5 Easy Breathing Exercises for Seniors Who Dislike Meditation. (n.d.). Www.seniorhelpers.com https://www.seniorhelpers.com/mi/grosse-pointe/resources/blogs/2023-05-11/

Antoine, C. (2023, April 6). The Role of Mindfulness in Achieving Fitness Goals. Lakeshore Sport & Fitness. https://lakeshoresf.com/the-role-of-mindfulness-in-achieving-fitness-goals/

Garone, S. (2023, December 18). How to Use Mindfulness to Achieve Your Nutrition and Fitness Goals. Verywell Fit. https://www.verywellfit.com/how-mindfulness-can-help-you-achieve-nutrition-and-fitness-goals-6825952

Juliano-Villani, G. (2023, January 9). Mindful Breathing: Definition, Techniques, & Benefits. Choosing Therapy. https://www.choosingtherapy.com/mindful-breathing/

McLeod, J. (2024, February 23). Stress Relief: Mindfulness Techniques for Seniors and Caregivers – All Seniors Care. All Seniors Care.

https://www.allseniorscare.com/stress-relief-mindfulness-techniques-for-seniors-and-caregivers/

Meyer, C. (2022, September 21). 10 Mindfulness Exercises & Activities for Older Adults. SWM. https://secondwindmovement.com/mindfulness-activities/

Rusinko, C. (2023, June 9). Mindful Drawing: Activities that Embrace Experimentation. Www.nga.gov. https://www.nga.gov/stories/mindful-drawing.html

spinutech. (2023a, September 20). 4 Simple Mindfulness Exercises for Seniors. Harbour's Edge. https://www.harboursedge.com/blog/health-wellness/4-simple-mindfulness-exercises-for-seniors/

spinutech. (2023b, September 20). 5 Mindfulness Exercises for Seniors. The Stayton. https://www.thestayton.com/blog/health-wellness/5-mindfulness-exercises-for-seniors/

12 gentle seated stretching exercises for seniors in 4 minutes. (2022, July 28). DailyCaring. https://dailycaring.com/12-easy-and-gentle-seated-stretching-exercises-for-seniors-in-4-minutes-video/

Chair yoga for seniors. (n.d.). Performancehealth.com. https://www.performancehealth.com/articles/chair-yoga-for-seniors-6-exercises-to-maintain-strength-and-flexibility

Lifestyle, S. (2020, February 12). Top 10 chair yoga positions for seniors [infographic]. Senior Lifestyle. https://www.seniorlifestyle.com/resources/blog/infographic-top-10-chair-yoga-positions-for-seniors/

Munuhe, N. (2022, August 16). Chair yoga for seniors: 10 poses to improve strength, flexibility, and balance. BetterMe Blog; BetterMe. https://betterme.world/articles/chair-yoga-for-seniors/

Alexander, B. (2015, November 16). 10 Relaxing Chair Yoga Exercises. Conscious Living TV. https://consciouslivingtv.com/bianca-alexander/blog/yoga/10-relaxing-chair-yoga-exercises.html

British Heart Foundation. (2019). 5 more easy chair exercises. Bhf.org.uk. https://www.bhf.org.uk/informationsupport/heart-matters-magazine/activity/chair-based-exercises/5-more-chair-based-exercises

Health, V. (2020, January 28). 18 Chair Exercises for Seniors & How to Get Started. Vive Health. https://www.vivehealth.com/blogs/resources/chair-exercises-for-seniors

Top 10 chair yoga positions for seniors [Infographic]. (2020, February 12). Senior Lifestyle. https://www.seniorlifestyle.com/resources/blog/infographic-top-10-chair-yoga-positions-for-seniors/

USA, H. (2018, March 1). 8 Effective Seated Exercises for Seniors in Wheelchairs. HUR USA - for LIFELONG STRENGTH. https://hurusa.com/8-effective-seated-exercises-for-wheelchair-bound-seniors/

Yoga exercises you can try at home. (n.d.). Www.bhf.org.uk. https://www.bhf.org.uk/informationsupport/heart-matters-magazine/activity/yoga/yoga-poses

Better Health Channel. (2012). Exercise - the low-down on hydration. Vic.gov.au. https://www.betterhealth.vic.gov.au/health/healthyliving/Exercise-the-low-down-on-water-and-drinks

CDC. (2021, January 25). Why It Matters. CDC. https://www.cdc.gov/nutrition/about-nutrition/why-it-matters.html

Ferreira, M. (2018). 6 Essential Nutrients: What They Are and Why You Need Them. Healthline. https://www.healthline.com/health/food-nutrition/six-essential-nutrients

Fletcher, J. (2019a, January 4). How to Eat a Balanced Diet: A Guide. Www.medicalnewstoday.com. https://www.medicalnewstoday.com/articles/324093

Fletcher, J. (2019b, August 22). 6 essential nutrients: Sources and why you need them. Www.medicalnewstoday.com. https://www.medicalnewstoday.com/articles/326132

Food, Drink, and Exercise – Top Tips for Nutrition and Hydration. (n.d.). Www.sunshinegym.co.uk. https://www.sunshinegym.co.uk/blog/articles/food-drink-exercise-nutrition-hydration.html

Green, S., & Shallal, K. (2020, August 23). Essential Nutrients. Open.maricopa.edu; Maricopa Community Colleges. https://open.maricopa.edu/nutritionessentials/chapter/essential-nutrients/

Harvard Health Publishing. (2019). Nutrition - Harvard Health. Harvard Health; Harvard Health. https://www.health.harvard.edu/topics/nutrition

Harvard T.H. Chan. (2017, September 28). The importance of hydration. News. https://www.hsph.harvard.edu/news/hsph-in-the-news/the-importance-of-hydration/

Krans, B. (2020, June 29). Balanced Diet: What Is It and How to Achieve It. Healthline. https://www.healthline.com/health/balanced-diet

Kyle Bradford Jones. (2017, March 27). Hydration: Why It's So Important - familydoctor.org. Familydoctor.org. https://familydoctor.org/hydration-why-its-so-important/

Lifestyle Desk. (2022, October 17). Optimise your post-workout nutrition for better recovery with these expert-approved tips. The Indian Express. https://indianexpress.com/article/lifestyle/health/post-workout-nutrition-tips-optimum-recovery-nutrients-hydration-timing-8208390/

Samaddar, R. (2022, January 24). Balanced Diet - Definition, Importance, Benefits & Diet Chart. Www.maxhealthcare.in. https://www.maxhealthcare.in/blogs/what-is-a-balanced-diet

Samuels, C. (2020, August 14). 20 Easy Recipes for Senior Nutrition. A Place for Mom. https://www.aplaceformom.com/caregiver-resources/articles/easy-recipes-for-senior-nutrition

The Cleaner Admin. (2021, June 2). The importance of good nutrition. Jamaica-Gleaner.com. https://jamaica-gleaner.com/article/health/20210602/importance-good-nutrition

Why Is It Important To Drink Water During Exercise | BRITA®. (n.d.). Www.brita.co.uk. https://www.brita.co.uk/news-stories/dispenser/drinking-water-during-exercise

Habit Formation. (2023, June 26). Psychology Today. https://www.psychologytoday.com/us/basics/habit-formation

Healthdirect Australia. (n.d.). How to improve your posture. Posture Exercises for Home and Work | Healthdirect. https://www.healthdirect.gov.au/how-to-improve-your-posture

Home, K. A. (n.d.). Eight (8) Simple Breathing Exercises for Older Adults. https://www.kendalathome.org/blog/breathe-easy-six-breath-exercises-for-older-adults

Precisionbiotics. (2023, October 16). The importance of forming good habits - PrecisionBiotics. Precision Biotics. https://www.precisionbiotics.co.uk/blog/mental-wellbeing/the-importance-of-forming-good-habits/

Solis-Moreira, J. (2024, January 9). Engaging your core is not the same as sucking in your belly. Here's the right way to do it. CNN. https://edition.cnn.com/2024/01/09/health/how-to-engage-your-core-wellness/index.html

Strong, R. (2022, September 19). Habits Matter More Than You Might Think — These Tips Can Help the Good Ones Stick. Healthline. https://www.healthline.com/health/mental-health/why-are-habits-important#professional-support

Wahome, C. (2021, August 20). 4 Benefits of Chair Exercises. WebMD. https://www.webmd.com/fitness-exercise/features/4-benefits-chair-exercises-seniors

Yanek, D. (1970, January 1). How to Engage Your Core During Any Type of Workout. https://www.onepeloton.com/blog/how-to-engage-your-core/

Made in United States
Orlando, FL
03 November 2024

53315156R00127